PSYCHOLOGY RESEARCH PROGRESS

PSYCHOLOGICAL SERVICE OF HIGHER EDUCATION INSTITUTIONS

PSYCHOLOGY RESEARCH PROGRESS

Additional books and e-books in this series can be found on Nova's website under the Series tab.

PSYCHOLOGY RESEARCH PROGRESS

PSYCHOLOGICAL SERVICE OF HIGHER EDUCATION INSTITUTIONS

SVITLANA V. KUCHERENKO
EDITOR

nova science publishers
New York

Library of Congress Cataloging-in-Publication Data

ISBN: 978-1-53618-160-9

Published by Nova Science Publishers, Inc. † New York

CONTENTS

INTRODUCTION

According to the Concept of psychological service development in the educational system in the Russian Federation until 2025, it is necessary to improve the psychological support of educational activities, taking into account new requirements for the psychological and pedagogical conditions for the implementation of educational programs. Among the urgent problems facing our psychological service of institutions of higher education is a decrease in the levels of mental and psychological health of the subjects of the educational process, an increase in gambling and Internet addictions, desocialization, victimization, the phenomena of violence and aggression, illegal students' actions, inter-ethnic tension, transnational conflicts etc.

So, the peculiarity of the students' and undergraduates' career anchors were studied by S. Kucherenko. Value-semantic orientations of students with Internet addiction is investigated by I. Sultanova and O. Shutova. Victimism, the phenomena of violence and illegal actions are not considered in the monograph, because the practice of the psychological service of the Humanitarian and Pedagogical Academy 2014-2019 has never come across anything like that.

The scientific novelty of the monograph lies in the fact that the need to provide psychological assistance to young people for successful socialization in the new social situation is considered comprehensively – in the unity of the theoretical and methodological foundations of the psychological service organization of the university and empirical research in each of the areas (psycho-diagnostic, psycho-correctional, psychological education and psychological counseling).

Modern scientific research ascertains the blurring and crisis of social identity, the growth of negative phenomena in the youth environment. Various risks are currently being updated: the growth of gaming and Internet addiction, desocialization, victimization, phenomena of violence, aggression (incident in Kerch), illegal actions and antisocial behavior of students; interethnic tension and interethnic conflicts, a decrease in tolerance in communication between people of different cultures. Such trends are associated, with the fact that the psychological services of educational institutions do not always pay attention to the solution and prevention of these problems.

The first chapter “Acmeological development of the university students” discusses the organization of the psychological services of a university (L. Bura and Ya. Zalevskaya). L. Bura examines successful adaptation of high school students as a necessary condition for their acmeological development. Psychological and acmeological development of the students’ personality in higher schools in the educational environment is considered in the theoretical study by E. Ponomareva, O. Rudakova.

The second chapter, “Research of the university psychological service” is devoted to the empirical aspects of psychological service of a university, exactly: career anchors of students and undergraduates (S. Kucherenko), the study of the attention parameters peculiarities and their dynamics in 17-23-year-old female students (E. Brunner), B. Hellinger’s systemic constellation as a method of research for an aesthetic object in the process of studying Art history (V. Vynohradov, E. Brunner), value-semantic orientations of students connected with Internet addiction (I. Sultanova, O. Shutova).

The third chapter “Directions of the university psychological service’ work” considers advanced psychological diagnostics of first-year students as a factor in the effectiveness of teaching at a university (M. Latysheva), psychological counseling as a line of work of a practical psychologist (I. Erina), educational activities in the system of psychological support of higher education (G. Grigoryev) and psychological correction of university students in the conditions of the Crimea's integration into the Russian socio-cultural space (O. Usatenko, M. Maik). The current Concept for the development of psychological service in the education system in the Russian Federation until 2025 provides for the provision of free psychological and pedagogical correction of personal development deficiencies for students.

The monograph presents the research of the Department of Psychology of Humanities and Education Science Academy in Yalta (branch) of the V. I. Vernadsky Crimean Federal University in Yalta for 2018-2019.

In: Psychological Service …
Editor: Svitlana V. Kucherenko
ISBN: 978-1-53618-160-9

Chapter 1

Acmeological Development of a Student at a University: Organization of the University Psychological Service

***Lyudmila V. Bura*[*], *PhD and Yana G. Zalevskaya*[†]**
Psychology Department,
V. I. Vernadsky Crimean Federal University, Crimea, Russia

Abstract

The Chapter deals with the issues of psychological support for personal and professional identification of students of psychology. It discusses major practice areas for the Counseling Center with the Department of Psychology. Long-term objectives are set for the implementation by the Counseling Center with the involvement of students and graduates of the Psychology Department. The main areas of the University Counseling Center practice are discussed.

[*] Corresponding Author's Email: buraselivanova.l@mail.ru.
[†] Corresponding Author's Email: ya.zalevskaya18@gmail.com.

Keywords: university counseling service, management, development areas, psychological problems of students

INTRODUCTION

Innovative processes taking place in higher education, the integration of students in the sociocultural space of the Russian Federation require a change in the educational paradigm to prepare a specialist who is competitive in the global labor market.

At the same time, the competitiveness of a graduate of a modern university requires not only professional knowledge, but also special abilities of the person, that provide her with the dynamism of professional behavior, new information search and assimilation independence, adequate solutions in "non-standard situations." Today, specialists who possess not only the appropriate qualifications, but also qualities such as: the ability to communicate with people, solve conflict situations, make innovative decisions, navigate in a new situation and adapt to new living conditions are more in demand (Grier-Reed 2012, 87). The formation of these qualities is a key task of a modern educational institution.

In order to form a productive professional position of a young specialist, it is necessary to provide social and psychological support to the student, as well as assistance in expanding his internal personal space, disclosing methods of self-knowledge, self-improvement, and reflection.

Therefore, at the present stage of the higher education system development, the professional development of students' psychological support, which is designed to improve the quality of their training as future specialists, seems relevant and necessary to us.

METHODS

Participants

Higher education is one of the most important links in the educational space for the formation of a specialist. We distinguish such components as the educational process, non-institutional forms of education (institute of curators, counselor school, affiliation, student clubs, etc.) in the educational space of the university. From our point of view, the psychological service should be one of the most important elements of the educational space (Bura 2016, 116).

By the educational space of a university, we mean a certain territory that is associated with large-scale phenomena in the field of education as a certain part of the social space within which normalized educational activities are carried out (Shegda 2018, 23).

The inclusion of a student in the educational space of a university goes through overcoming the personality problems of a future specialist. This process is designed to accompany the psychological service.

The main types of work of a psychologist in the education system are: diagnosis, correction, rehabilitation, prevention, psychological education.

Today the Russian Federation has already some experience in implementing assistance to participants in the educational process in higher educational institutions, but the problem is that the experience of psychological service in a university is small and practically duplicates the psychological service in a secondary school, without taking into account the specifics of higher education. Therefore, the psychological service of the university requires certain reorganization.

In addition to students, the participants in the educational process are also teachers, job seekers, graduate students, administration, teaching and support staff, which also need psychological support, since the existing system of advanced training of specialists is not able to solve the whole range of tasks facing it (Lin and Huang 2014, 77).

So, there is a need for a holistic approach to providing psychological support to all participants in the educational process of the university. We believe that the psychological service is designed to ensure the realization of the personal, professional, creative potential of the individual, create conditions for self-realization of the personality, and provide psychological support to all subjects of educational activity.

From our point of view, the psychological service is called upon, first of all, to form the psychological readiness of the participants in the educational process for professional activities. Its goal should be to help students to realize their personal qualities, reflection, creating conditions for the development of personality.

In addition, the psychological service can significantly affect the formation of professional identity of students, their personal growth, the development of leadership qualities, communication skills and the like.

N. Chepeleva in her studies identifies the following areas of the psychological service at the university:

- psycho-prophylactic work among students and teachers;
- psycho-diagnostic work among students;
- psycho-correctional work among students (in case of insufficient psycho-prophylactic work and, if necessary, timeliness and effectiveness of the application of psycho-correction methods and general psychotherapy);
- advisory work commissioned by students and teachers;
- educational work to clarify current problems and methods of psychology (Chepeleva and Povyakel 2001, 65).

The results of the monitoring indicate that the development of the psychological service in higher education institutions has been stepped up, but at the same time, they also emphasize that this is not enough and that there is no single, well-defined structural and functional organization of such a service. There are various organizational forms of psychological support at a university: the position of a psychologist; psychological center; psychological laboratory; psychological office; psychological service; psychological sector; group of practical psychology; psychological consultation; psychological department and the like in Russia. But the number of psychological services in universities, at the moment, is very small. At most universities, the urgent needs for psychological support of the educational process are met by scientific and pedagogical staff in the absence of adequate funding and material and technical support on a volunteer basis, which is caused by the urgent need for this (Shkarlet and Gorshunova 2018, 20).

The results of the analysis of information from university reports indicate that there are almost no rates of social educators in the psychological services of universities, partly the functions of social educators are performed by practical psychologists, and the socio-pedagogical support of the educational process is not carried out in full - only certain types of work with limited number of students, in the absence of methodological and material and technical support (Prince 2015, 5).

The instructive recommendations on the activities of psychological service workers emphasize that special attention should be paid to the selection and creation of the most effective forms and methods of individual and group work of the university's psychological service with students and teachers (psycho-preventive and psycho-hygienic, diagnostic, consulting, developmental and correctional techniques) aimed at self-development, self-actualization and self-realization of the individual, designed to contribute to the process of social-psychological adaptation of students, and it is noted that universities need special assistance:

- organizational and normative (documentary definition of the organizational and functional structure of the psychological service and the status of its employees);
- financial (identification and provision of sources of financing and material and technical support for the activities of the psychological service);
- scientific and methodological (providing scientific and methodological recommendations regarding the forms, methods and content of the activities of practical psychologists and social educators);

- informational (exchange of best practices and innovative technologies, organization of scientific and practical conferences and seminars).

Obviously, the necessity to create and further develop the psychological service at the university is caused by problems in the system of professional higher education, in particular, in the formation of the personality of a professional. In addition, during the study and discussion of educational technologies (unity of goals, content and teaching methods), the need for didactic correspondence not only to their subject content, but also to the psychological, social and personal characteristics of future specialists is clearly recognized. Modern society has really come across the fact that the professional training of students cannot be limited to only strict professional orientation components. A comprehensive development of the competency-based approach is necessary, an integral part of which is the creation of conditions for the full-fledged personal development of specialists.

Particularly urgent is the problem of creating psychological services in technical universities, especially in those ones, where there is no department of psychology. However, students of these institutions have the same problems as students of the humanitarian profile. Moreover, it is possible that in technical universities a psychological service is more needed, because if a humanities student in its absence can seek an advice of a psychologist or a teacher, then students of technical universities are deprived of this.

Systematic, focused work of specialists of the psychological service of a technical university will reduce the severity of students' problems. Training sessions to adapt to the group, to the educational institution, individual and group consultations, psychological prevention should be conducted for students of all specialties, including technical ones. Psychologists can advise students on self-organization and time planning, psychological readiness for the session and behavior on the exam, teach relaxation and self-regulation techniques, help to cope with emotional difficulties during the adaptation period, solve problems of interpersonal relationships and communication in student groups. Moreover, the psychological service can greatly help technical teachers (seminars, trainings, etc.).

In order for such psychological services to be created and developed, it is necessary to conduct studies to generalize and analyze the existing experience of their work in domestic and foreign universities, determine the methodological foundations, the concept of the psychological service, and create an appropriate legal framework. But, despite the fact that the problematic circle of organization of a psychological service in a university is still not well defined, now, taking into account the experience of the psychological service in other social spheres, we can outline the methodological and strategic guidelines for the activity of such a service in the educational space of a university.

The methodology of the organization of the psychological service at the university should contain:

- a set of scientific and theoretical principles of its functioning (which should determine whether such a service can realize strategic functions in the process of modernization of higher education);
- fixed assets (technological, personnel, other resources with which its goals and objectives will be solved);
- methods of work of psychologists;
- key rules of activity, etc.

The theory of developmental psychology, development objectives and the dominant motivation of student youth are the methodological foundations of the psychological services of the university. Theoretical analysis and extensive experimental studies show that the age of students is the age of solving the problems of development and implementation of functions that lie not only in the field of professional training. The profession is acquired in order to be realized as a person, to ensure a decent life for oneself, to start a family, and determine one's life prospects.

On the one hand, modern society imposes a moratorium for youth to search for themselves and self-determination; on the other hand, it offers a fairly adequate and constructive image of the future and its meaning. This situation can have an extremely negative impact on determining the direction of the personal development of subjects of the educational space. An ideal image of the future includes an idea of a professional and career line of development, family relationships, the desire for self-development. This is not a complete list of age-related tasks of the psychological development of student youth. It is impossible to ignore all these features in the organization of higher education. The dominant needs of students must be addressed. It is necessary to get rid of the illusions that the educational, cognitive needs of students can minimize the motivation of the dominant tasks of age. Failure to understand this can aggravate the contradictions between the motivational mood of young people and the demands of teachers.

The main areas of work of the psychological service of the university in motivational aspects of student life:

- resolving the contradictions between the dominant necessity of youth and ignoring them by organizational structures of the university;
- elimination of the illusions of teachers on the dominant motivational basis of students' educational activities;
- psychological justification of the requirements for creating the optimal coordination between solving age-related problems of student life and the process of vocational training.

Student age is called the peak phase of the development of logical thinking, creative imagination, intuition, arbitrary selectivity of knowledge, semantic integrity and awareness. But, unfortunately, due to the circumstances of the ongoing reform of school education, some students have obvious gaps, shortcomings, imbalances in the development of the cognitive sphere (for example, in the types of perception, thinking, imagination, memory). Such students need the qualified help of a psychologist for a successful professional determination. These problems should be solved by the psychological service of the university.

The main areas of work of the psychological service of the university on the intellectual development of students are as follows:

- research work;
- individual counseling;
- work on the development of the cognitive sphere of students;
- addressing the shortcomings of the cognitive processes of individual students (by means of group trainings for the development of creativity of thinking, etc.).

The modern psychological service of the university is a radically new service. The new psychological service of the university is an integrated system that should combine the main structural components: psychological diagnostics (individual and group), counseling, psychological prevention, promotion of psychological knowledge, socio-psychological adaptation of students in educational and professional activities, raising their spiritual level development and psychological culture, training sessions, seminars, conferences and the like.

In our opinion, the approximate structure of the psychological service at the university should include the following elements: a psychological assistance center (for personal problems); center for psychological games and psycho-training; center for psychological education; research and psycho diagnostic centers.

A questionnaire of students showed that they see the functions of the psychological service of the university in adapting to new learning conditions, including the conditions of a credit-modular system, solving problems with teachers, assistance to young families, solving personal problems, self-knowledge and assistance in finding employment and adapting to professional activities. Psychological students and social educators note the need for practical activity as experience; therefore they offer themselves as volunteers or trainees of this service.

Of course, we cannot consider student models as independent and scientifically based ones, but conducting surveys contributed to the awareness of the problems of the psychological service, its function and place in the educational space of the university. In the process of our activities, we developed a model of the university's psychological service for the implementation in the Humanities and Education Science Academy (branch) of V. I. Vernadsky Crimean Federal University in Yalta.

The presented model of the university's psychological service contains the following areas: work with students (internships by students as psychologists and social educators on the basis of the service by order of the student and administration, social and psychological support), work with employers (social and psychological support of the graduate, advanced training, order).

The outlined circle of questions allows us to draw the following conclusions:

1. At the present stage of development of the higher education system, the psychological support of the professional development of students is relevant and necessary; it will increase the quality of their training as future specialists. In addition, there is a need for a holistic approach to providing psychological support to all participants in the educational process of the university.
2. Today in the Russian Federation there is already some experience in implementing assistance to participants of the educational process in higher education, but this experience is small and practically duplicates the psychological service in a secondary educational institution, without taking into account the specifics of higher education. Therefore, the psychological service of the university requires certain reorganization and the creation of a regulatory, methodological base for the activities of the psychological service of universities.
3. The solution to this problem may be the organization and realization of the All-Russian experiment on the development and

testing of various models of the psychological service of the university.

4. The presented model of the psychological service of the university for implementation in the Humanitarian and Pedagogical Academy is one of the ways to solve the problem.

The prospect of further research, we see the testing of this model and monitoring its work.

Thus, the psychological service of the university is a promising area for interaction and mutual enrichment of theory and practice, psychological assistance and support of the development of a future professional.

References

Bura L. V. 2016. “The psychological service of the university: problems and prospects” *Gumanitarnye nauki* [*Humanitarian sciences*]. 1. P. 116.

Chepeleva N. V. and Povyakel N. I. 2001 “Psychological service in higher educational institutions” *Prakticheskaya psihologiya i social’naya rabota* [*Practical Psychology and Social Work*]. 6 (33). P. 65.

Grier-Reed T. 2012 “Exploring the Student Engagement Instrument and Career Perceptions with College Students” *Journal of Educational and Developmental Psychology*. 2. PP. 85-96.

Lin Sh. H. and Huang Y. Ch. 2014 “Life Stress and Academic Burnout” *Active Learning in Higher Education*. 15 (1). PP. 77-90.

Prince J. P. 2015 “University student counseling and mental health in the United States: Trends and challenges” *Mental Health & Prevention*. 3(1-2). P. 5-10.

Shegda O. V. 2018 “Psychological service as an element of the educational space of the university” *Aktual’nye problemy psihologii* [*Actual problems of psychology*]. 7. P. 23.

Shkarlet S. M. and Gorshunova I. V. 2018 "Innovative development of educational space in higher educational institutions" *Vestnik Chernigovskogo gosudarstvennogo tekhnologicheskogo universiteta* [*Bulletin of Chernihiv State Technological University*]. 2. P. 20.

In: Psychological Service …
Editor: Svitlana V. Kucherenko
ISBN: 978-1-53618-160-9

Chapter 2

Acmeological Development of a Student at a University: Psychological and Acmeological Development of the Students' Personality in Higher Schools in the Educational Environment

Elena Y. Ponomareva**, *PhD and Olga A. Rudakova
Psychology Department,
V. I. Vernadsky Crimean Federal University, Crimea, Russia

Abstract

The chapter is devoted to the main problems and features of the acmeological development of the personality of the future psychologist, the means of forming their professional competence. Theoretical research is aimed at finding ways to solve the problems of psychological and acmeological development of future specialists, whereby to realize the

* Corresponding Author's Emails: astra.59@bk.ru; grin-lief@mail.ru.

acquired potential in the process of preparation for professional activity. And also, an attempt is made to systematize the criteria and mechanisms of the acmeological development of the personality as an independent process, which is a multi-stage and level process of the self-realization of the personality in activities on the path to achieving “acme”.

Keywords: “acme”, acmeology, personality, psychologist, development, psychological and acmeological

INTRODUCTION

Today, the changes that Russian society is undergoing in the social, economic, cultural and political space affect psychological processes in all social groups, and we can observe a special reflection of these processes among students. Behavioral patterns of students studying in higher education institutions are determined by social status (status), as well as characteristic qualities and psychosocial properties that are distinctive in relation to a given socio group, such as mental mobility, IQ mobility, the prevalence of emotionality over rationalism, etc.

Thus, modern psychology raises questions about the socio-psychological regulation of the behavior of studying youth in higher educational establishments, the assimilation of socially significant norms by them, as well as the psychological and acmeological development of their personality, which is especially important, since namely young professionals represent the basis for the formation of the next stage in the formation of society in the socio-cultural space of the Russian Federation (Rudakova O.A. 2019).

Based on the legislative framework in the field of higher education of the Russian Federation, which sets the goals of social and state order for higher education, and this is the provision of quality education, which is reflected in accordance with the federal state educational standard of higher education. federal state educational standard for the training of highly qualified personnel in postgraduate school and federal state requirements, and it is also significant that the customer has educational services and the demand for these specialists.

Today, it remains important, for the scientific community in the field of psychology and acmeology, to solve the following problematic issues (Rudakova O.A. 2019):

1) The study, testing and implementation of psychological and acmeological research in the field of personality development of students in higher education is explained by the fact that this age is an important period in the process of becoming a future professional. Awareness of the goals and meaning of life, the formation of professional competencies, the formation of sustainable worldviews etc. are extremely important. We consider the issue, partially reflected in the writings of such scientists as G. Abramova, V. Alekseeva, E. Volkova, B. Kruglova, I Kulagina, A. Mudrik, A. Safina, A. Tolstykh, D. Feldstein, E. Spranger. Most of the scientists presented believe that the age we are considering is sensitive for the formation of our own worldview based on strong beliefs, attitudes and the ability to independently model and predict our individual life path. The relevance of the problems of studying the psychological and acmeological development of the personality of students in higher education is substantiated by the socio-cultural reorganization of the society. Thus, as a prelude to "alternative scenarios" of the personal development of students in higher education, including the dissemination of antisocial values, beliefs and ideas of various youth subcultures, we see the effective implementation of programs, techniques and methods based on acmeo-psychological research.
2) The search for ways, methods, means and techniques of effective personal development in the context of a mobile, innovative and active professional, receptive to environmental reforms and aimed at self-realization of personal potential in the changing socio-cultural space of the state. This issue is relevant and is studied in modern studies of acmeologists, such as A. Derkach, V.Zazykin,

N.Koval, N. Kuzmina, A. Markova, E. Saiko, I. Semenov, Y. Sinyagin. and others. According to the opinion of most scientists, the presented trend depends on the process of "humanization of the human sciences" and the substitution of basic priorities in the paradigm of acmeology. Scientific research, in particular, is focused on the person and does not affect his professional or sociocultural phenomena in general. In whatever group we consider "personality," it is always the subject of its development; in other words, it determines the totality of the processes of self-actualization, self-realization, self-regulation and self-improvement, which is essentially the main task of acmeology.

3) Search for ways to optimize the process of personality development, including acmeological. This problem field has a scientific backlog in the studies of leading acmeologists, such as: S. Alekseev, A. Asmolov, I. Vachkov, M. Dmitriev, O. Kachanova., V. Kolbanov, V. Kulganov, Y. Parfenov, V. Rybnikov etc. We see the goal, to optimize the psychological and acmeological development of the personality of students in higher education in the context of integration into the socio-cultural field of Russian society. The main task, in our opinion, is the search for new methods, techniques, methods and models of psychological and acmeological development of a competitive, adaptive and comprehensively developed personality in Russian society.

METHODS

Participants

Acmeology today is a fairly young direction, while it has the experience of theoretical and practical research in the vector of personality development. Questions of the construction itself, as well as the methodological and technological support of the acmeological development of the personality of students mastering professionally-oriented activities in various areas of Russian society are raised in the studies of such scientists as: O. Anisimova, V. Agapova, A. Gusev, S. Kandybovich, A. Kirichenko, R. Krichevsky, O.Moskalenko, E. Klimova, A. Markova, A. Ogneva, E. Selezneva, Y. Sinyagina, L. Stepnova.

Since acmeology is aimed at solving the problems of personal and professional development of future specialists through the development of effective models, methods and techniques that allow realizing the acquired potential by a person in the process of preparation for professional activity, therefore, in scientific papers of A. Derkach and E. Saiko, increased attention is paid to this. Scientists have revealed that the basis of the acmeological development of the personality as an independent process is a multi-stage and level process of self-realization of an individual in an activity, during which a cyclic phenomenon occurs, leading simultaneously to the formation of a need for a new activity, at a different level, varying in structure, content, in degree severity and security (Derkach A.A. and Sajko E.V. 2009; Klimov E.A. 1995).

An analysis of the theoretical and methodological foundations of the issue under study allows us to conclude that at the moment the question of the concept of "acmeological development of the personality of students in the student period" remains open and the psychological and acmeological essence of the development of students the personality-forming factors in higher education is not fully covered.

Thanks to the activities of scientists such as A. Derkach, N. Kuzmin, O. Moskalenko, E. Saiko and L. Fursi.the term "acmeological personality development" is widely used in the framework of acmeology and developmental psychology, and K. Petrov and N. Soloviev use it in pedagogy. At the same time, there are not enough works revealing the acmeological development of the personality of students in higher education as combining a personality's resource that can be empirically observed, measured, scientifically designed and developed in higher educational institutions, and this is a significant range of both theoretical and empirical studies.

A content analysis of the works of domestic and foreign scientists allows us to conclude that the phenomenon we are considering, such as the acmeological development of the personality of students in higher education, appears in a real educational environment. At the moment, psychology and acmeology of the education system should have a goal to improve the set of personal and socio-professional qualities of future specialists in the context of the socio-cultural space of the Russian Federation.

The presented goal reflects the essence of discrepancies between social aspirations and the requirements presented by the sociological and cultural environment for modern youth: creativity and initiative, creative independence and enterprise, responsibility and personal and professional competence, as well as inconsistency between the tasks of the educational system, i.e., implementation of the humanistic educational paradigm.

In terms of the acmeological development of the personality of students in higher education, the presented discrepancy is exacerbated by a number of more particular contradictions, namely: between the relevance of the research topic and the undeveloped methodological basis of the psychological and acmeological phenomenon; between the need for the formation of the basic components of students psychological and acmeological personality development and the lack of technologies, methods and programs, as well as the holistic concept of the acmeological personality development of students in higher educational institutions of the Russian Federation.

The need to resolve these discrepancies determines the relevance of our chosen topic. In connection with the noted discrepancies, there is a research issue that proceeds from the need for a holistic concept of acmeological development of the personality of students in higher education, in which you can systematically implement the acmeological approach, which combines the key provisions of such concepts as personality-oriented, humanistic, pragmatic, etc (Luk'yanova M.I. 2014).

Due to the fact that the age period under consideration, such as students, is basic in the process of formation and development of the personality of a future specialist, since, at this age, according to the main periodizations of mental development, a moral stable component of the personality actively develops. In their actions, students of higher education are based on their own foundations and views, values and attitudes that are formed on the "platform" of life experience and are associated with the establishment of a more or less holistic worldview, therefore the acmeological concept, combined with the approaches included in it, provides a systematic study of the problem of acmeological personal development of students in your high school.

The personal and professional formation of students in higher educational institutions is accompanied by the process of accumulation and systematization of general cultural and professional knowledge, an increase in interest in oneself and others, it should also be pointed out that the basis for the formation of worldview views is the development of reflection as the main neoplasm of a given age. There is a search for clear answers, categorical views are formed. It is reflected in certain dogmatism in relation to specific life situations, in other words, they still have teenage maximalism (Luk'yanova M.I. 2014).

These processes are important for the future specialist, since the worldview correlates with the solution of semantic problems, such as social orientation, self-awareness as a unit of a social group, social status and position when choosing future path and ways to achieve goals. So, this age period, is the time of solving the fundamental problems of personal-social self-determination, which precedes the entry into an independent professional life-activity in accordance with a particular opportunity and personality abilities.

To date, the majority of scientists consider personal self-determination as a basic psychological neoplasm of the age, at this stage of life it is important that within the framework of the formation of this level of self-consciousness, a relatively stable idea of oneself existed, that is, the self-concept (Luk'yanova M.I. 2014).

Due to the fact that future specialists at a higher educational institution solve not only a large number of professional tasks, but mainly designed to provide effective functioning of educational and cognitive activities, the main resource of personal and professional formation is the definition of primary, personally significant educational and cognitive tasks and coordination goals aimed at mastering future professional activities. In this process, the orientation of the personality of students towards academic and professional performance ceases to be the over-target, but becomes one of the positions of the personality-professional formation. The student acquires a set of methods for transferring knowledge into a tool for solving substantive, technical, personal, implementation and professional tasks.

Based on the foundation of the ideas of acmeology of education, we can state the possibility of developing the personality of students in higher education in the process of assimilation of their future profession.

So, the concept of "acmeological development" in the pedagogical sphere is quite new, since the conceptual field of this field of knowledge is insufficiently developed, therefore, the understanding of the essence of the mechanisms and content of the acmeological development of the personality of students in higher education is contradictory and now there is no certainty and unity in statements.

So, according to V. Maksimov's ideas of developing the concept of acmeological school education, the concept we study is described only from the perspective of the teacher and is typified as a derivative concept of the teacher's professional, personal and spiritual development. The concept of acme is formulated from the perspective of a humanistic attitude towards the achievement of success and good health of each specific subject of pedagogical activity, the development of the creative potential of both the teacher and the student in the process of their joint activity (Maksimova V.N. 2002).

N. Poletaeva determines "acmeological personality development" in the context of striving for achievements of high results, including both one's own pedagogical activity and the improvement of creative professional activity as a whole. This setting leads to a continuous search for new ways, techniques and methods aimed at creating innovative teaching technologies, to the development of new non-stereotypical ways to carry out professional activities, to objective self-esteem and reflection (Poletaeva N.M. 2014). According to the scientist, the acmeological development is the result of the value and ideological self-determination of the personality, aimed at life-forming strategies, such as health, life success and spirituality, which in turn forms the core of the social and valeological maturity of the individual.

Acmeology is not only the main direction of the psychology of personality development, but also acts as a worldview position, which reflects in the aggregate stable relations to the world, people and lifestyle. The acmeological position simultaneously acts as a result, and as an achievement of the personality, forms a unified layer of further development of the personality, manifesting itself as a potential force and at the same time accumulates and expresses the totality of life values of the personality and its basic needs for future life (Glinskij A.S. 2006).

A. Glinsky, in the concept of "acmeology" puts a combination of personal qualities of a professional orientation, contributing to personal and professional achievements and allowing achieving "acme". The scientist presents the student's acmeology as a combination of his current life meanings, dominant motives of activity, educational motivation, abilities and skills of educational activity, which is a leading activity in youth along with a communicative one (Glinskij A.S. 2006).

From the point of view of A. Derkach, who considers personal self-determination, that is, an already held statement of his own position in problematic personal situations, in its main characteristics:

- as a process of overcoming the mental gap between the current state and the need for self-realization;
- as a two-vector process of re-evaluating the manifestation of "I" in the situations of achieving a higher personal meaning and from higher personal meanings to methods of their objectification (Derkach A.A. and Sajko E.V. 2009).

Acmeological development can be expressed in the context of a subjective, meaningful attitude to certain life values, to activity, to a future profession, to cognition, which will be stable regulators of life and behavior of students in higher education.

It should be noted that psychological and acmeological support can have a tremendous impact on the development of the acmeological position of the student, on the personality development in general, the formation of worldview and professionalization.

The acmeological development of the personality of a student in higher education is largely connected with the psychological characteristics of the personality and is inconceivable out of society. In this regard, the process of forming the acmeological position of students has two qualitative manifestations:

1. The social position is determined by the system of relations that characterizes the behavioral style of the individual.
2. The position is personal-psychological, characterized by the views, perceptions and attitudes of the personality to the conditions of his own life, realized and defended by the personality in the reference groups at the stage of university education.

In the educational activity of a higher educational institution, in preparing future specialists in the process of interaction between the subjects of this process, acmeological development of a person should be considered in the unity of subjective and objective in a person, in addition, it is necessary to take into account the attitude to real values that affect goal setting, focus, choice of paths and means of their implementation. Since in situations of the educational process the student faces the necessity for free and independent choice, the inevitability of taking responsibility for their actions in the process of mastering the future profession, it is the choice itself that is a manifestation of the activity and personality of the individual. At the same time, it must be understood that not all students in higher education possess the techniques and means to accomplish this activity and show individuality, since the choice of means and actions is determined not only by the goals that the future specialist has set for himself, but also by circumstances and objective conditions. The student is faced with the task of confirming himself in the educational space as an individual and a personality, choosing, and, what is most important, defending his position. In this case it is important for him to be constantly ready for such a choice and capable of action, which is the key to the effectiveness of future professional activities.

In our opinion, the psychological and acmeological development of the personality acts as the key to determining the ability of students to carry out activities to master the future profession, this desire for achievement determines the role and place of the student, both in higher educational and in social cultural space of the Russian Federation and involves the "cultivation" of a value and responsible attitude to any activity, including his future professional one.

Thus, the acmeological component in the development of the personality of students is the process of forming an acmeological position, in other words, it is the readiness of a young specialist in any possible educational, personal or professional situation for action aimed at self-determination, achievements in the social, personal and educational fields. Further it will be possible to determine his internal activity and desire to achieve "highest achievements" in future professional activities (Bodalev A.A. 1998).

In our opinion, it is also necessary to turn to a problematic issue, such as determining the nature, structure, and functional characteristics of the acmeological position of students in higher educational institutions.

According to N. Borytko, to determine the functions of educational phenomena, such as personality, in the process of development and human life means to determine the role that is aimed at ensuring this phenomenon in human life as an integral being (Borytko N.M. 2005). So, studying the system of functions, the essence of the object being studied is revealed and it makes it possible to most fully characterize the psychological and acmeological development of the student's personality as an important task of his professional and personal formation.

N. Borytko emphasizes that in the field of sciences studying the socio-pedagogical aspect of human activity, function is understood to a greater extent as a qualitative characteristic aimed at maintaining, and developing the entire stable system. The constancy of the functional components of the system is determined by their relationship with the structural components of the personality and correlate with each other. The absence of such connections between the components leads to their isolation and subsequently to displacement from the system (Borytko N.M. and Mackajlova O.A. 2002; Borytko N.M. 2005).

Analyzing the essential characteristics of the acmeological development of the personality, as well as their importance in the personal and professional development of students in higher education, it is possible to distinguish such functions as self-esteem, self-understanding, self-affirmation, self-development and self-realization.

The function of self-esteem in the psychological and acmeological direction of the personality development of students in higher education is manifested through the students' awareness of personal cognitive processes, mental properties and conditions, the establishment of an adequate level of claims to themselves and their activities, as well as the comparison of their own achievements with the merits of others. Since self-esteem is the leading psychological factor in the formation of students' activities, it influences the formation of individual characteristics and age characteristics. Among the factors that determine the formation of self-regulation mechanisms, self-esteem is a central one and it determines the orientation and level of an individual's activity, the formation of his value orientations, personal meanings and, ultimately, "acme" achievements.

The function of self-esteem is comparable with the development of a reflexive function at a given age. Other functions, such as self-affirmation, subjectivity, and the acmeological position of a person in relation to his own development, are not possible without correlating oneself, one's meanings with the circumstances of the outside world, with sociocultural values, which is manifested in self-esteem. N. Borytko, like most scientists, considers self-esteem as an assessment by the subject of himself, his abilities, professional qualities and role in the creative transformation of himself and surrounding circumstances (Borytko N.M. and Mackajlova O.A. 2002; Borytko N.M. 2005). Due to the fact that self-esteem is a central component of the "I-concept" which manifests itself in the totality of self-images, the level of self-esteem reflects the degree of self-esteem and the nature of the orientation of the actions of students in higher education.

Within the framework of pedagogical acmeology, such researchers as A. Derkach., N. Kuzmina, A. Rean turn to such components of self-esteem as self-assessment of the achieved result and self-assessment of the potential of their capabilities. The first structure reflects satisfaction or dissatisfaction with one's own achievements, and the second one reflects faith in one's own strengths, in the ability to realize one's plans and intentions, and build one's perspective. Thus, a low achievement rate in combination with an overestimated self-esteem can become a leading factor in acmeological development, provided the student is personally interested and there is an effective psychological and acmeological method of influence.

Due to the fact that the personality's acmeological potential, as well as self-esteem, are manifested in the conditions of activity, the self-esteem structure can be represented in the form of self-esteem of the individual's potential, in other words, it is the implementation of an activity with the goal of achieving success or "acme", and it determines the strategies for realization of the set goals and objectives, the existence of the process of activity, that is, in what ways goals are achieved and tasks are realized; and the last one is the result and assimilation of what has been achieved (Rudakova O.A. 2019).

The function of self-understanding in the structure of the acmeological development of the personality of university students comes from the position of "self-affirmation", namely, understanding the meaning of personal life and the acmeological position as systems of dominant value-semantic relations.

According to V. Puzko self-understanding reveals itself as the creative potential of a person, which manifests itself in the appropriation and development of personal meanings, and is the result of a strenuous effort to exist in a derivative defense against the hidden manipulation of the sociocultural crisis. According to the scientist the purpose of self-understanding is the appropriation of personal meaning in the language of tradition, prejudice as the main forms of cultural and historical experience, it is manifested in behavioral patterns, in the internal dialogue in relation to the experience of the "other" to itself (Puz'ko V. I. 2003). Thus, the goal of self-understanding is not only the appropriation of the meaning of "I" in internal dynamics, but also the awareness of the subject in areas outside of himself, the phenomenal field and the surrounding reality.

According to U. Habermas, self-understanding in the acmeological paradigm is expressed in the process of developing the personality's ability to create an "individual life project" (Habermas, Yu. 2001), that is, to compose and realize one's life path. According to V. Mikhailov and T. Snegirev self-understanding is a definition of oneself in the field of professional and personal characteristics, which will allow a student in higher education to switch to a change of his internal position, to develop his identity (Luk'yanova M.I. 2014).

Due to the fact that self-understanding includes a category of meaning, which is considered in the context of personality subjectivity in a culture that forms in the student's personality, such components as values, meanings, norms, knowledge. The personal meaning of self-understanding is possible due to the active work of human consciousness. These personal components of self-understanding in connection with cultural characteristics cannot be assimilated by the student's personality, they develop, open as a result of an individual search, as a result of internal work, due to a person's own activity.

Acmeological development cannot be carried out without such a function of self-understanding as the reflective mental activity of the personality.

V. Andreev comes to the conclusion that education goes into self-education, upbringing into self-upbringing, learning into self-education, socialization into self-realization, provided that the person actively masters the philosophical, psychological and pedagogical culture, that is, becomes a philosopher, a psychologist, and a teacher for himself (Andreev V.I. 2015). This statement of the scientist shows the relationship between the function of self-understanding and the function of "acme", which is similar to the works of E. Borisova (Borisova E.V. 2006). It can be defined as "the subject's universal ability to identify, disclose and objectify its essential forces." Thus, acmeological development appears in the form of a stable orientation of the personality of students in higher education to demonstrate their creative strengths, their potential in the context of their own "acme".

At the same time, self-understanding of an individual's personality is closely connected with his self-affirmation, which subsequently leads to self-realization of his own "acme" potential.

The function of self-affirmation in the system of personality development of a student in higher education is determined by the leading need for self-esteem, self-affirmation in the eyes of the society and in one's own eyes. It is important for the individual to acquire certain properties that are valuable for personal and professional development as a whole and enter the sociocultural space of the Russian Federation. Due to the fact that the need for self-affirmation gives educational activities to students in higher education, it allows the formation of an individual character of the personality of a future specialist.

N. Borytko and O. Matskaylova, in their studies indicate that self-affirmation is self-awareness and attitude towards oneself, presentation of one's "concrete I" to other people, for whom it acts as an object. So, it turns out that such a presentation of your "concrete I" is manifested in certain strategies of behavior aimed at satisfying the student's desires for a high external assessment and self-esteem of his personality. In modern psychological and pedagogical literature, it is customary to distinguish three strategies of self-affirmation, and they are self-suppression, constructive self-assertion and domination (Borytko N.M. and Mackajlova O.A. 2002).

In the context of the acmeological position of the personality development of students in higher education, the function of self-affirmation has cause-effect relationships with the strategy of constructive self-affirmation. It allows us to consider self-affirmation as the achievement of subjective satisfaction with the result and the process of self-realization, that is, the implementation of "acme". Thus, the student in the process of realizing his personal and professional abilities strives to achieve a high level of social assessment and be competitive in the context of self-realization, according to the subjective standards defined by him.

According to Asmolov A.G. and Petrovsky A.V., self-affirmation manifests itself as the most important component of motivational-volitional regulation of the learner's personality, so when problematic and difficult situations arise on the path to self-realization, the learner does not resort to conformity, but on the contrary shows a desire to overcome difficulties.

The self-affirmation function activates the entire system of internal personal meanings and its development will be reflected in the following psychological-acmeological position, which involves:

- an individual level of socially active work, actualization of one's own intrapersonal potential, achievement of success in certain types of activity, overcoming of problem tasks and problems in mastering future professional activity;
- emotional-volitional regulation of the future specialist's behavior, directing his activity to the realization of potential opportunities and an emotive idea of the process of self-realization and expected success;
- reflection that allows you to analyze your goals, ways and opportunities to achieve them, adequately assess the results of activities, the attitude of others around them.

The acmeological position in the context of the personality development of students in higher education realizing the function of self-affirmation develops and strengthens the responsibility of the individual, since this function determines the nature of the student's interaction with the outside world in the process of performing various types of activities and allows you to consciously approach the development of a future profession.

The acmeological function of self-affirmation leads to successful self-development of a person, since this function ensures the implementation of the entire system of acmeological personality development in higher educational institutions, and this is personal, professional and social growth of a future specialist (Luk'yanova M.I. 2014).

There are a sufficient number of studies in psychological literature that consider self-development as a driving force of personal growth when achieving "acme". A halt in self-development leads to maladaptation due to changes in the surrounding socio-political and cultural space of the country. It should also be noted that this stop provokes the inability of the individual to receive and effectively use new knowledge and technologies, to solve professional and personal problems adequately, it is a significant limitation in the subjective formation of any person.

According to N. Peshkova the acmeological development of personality is embodied in the function of self-development through the manifestation of the following characteristics of the subject (Peshkova, N.A. 2012):

- the student is responsible for his own actions and for his further development;
- the student achieves success in those activities that appear for him the sphere of self-expression;
- the student receives satisfaction from the process of setting and subsequent solving new problems, includingone or another activity;
- the student seeks to gain a new life experience.

Studies of such scientists as O. Gazman, B. Vulfova, V. Ivanova and N. Sergeyev, allow us to conclude that self-development is an obligatory component of modern training of specialists, in terms of an indicator of personality subjectivity in the process of professional training. Self-development as a component of the acmeological development of the personality of students in higher education is closely related to such socio-psychological processes as goal setting, reflection, interaction with society, and self-regulation (Bodalev A.A. 1998; Turgunbayeva, B. 2013).

The function of self-realization in the process of acmeological development of the personality is manifested in its characteristics such as independence, freedom, creativity. In other words, self-realization lies in the student's ability to plan, regulate, set goals in relation to the activity itself, autonomously, by means of volitional efforts, carry out self-regulation of behavior, not excluding intersubjective interactions, as well as concentrate creative potential, be creative and independent in opinions and activities, be responsible for his actions and deeds (Peshkova, N.A. 2012). Moreover, such scientists as T. Bauer, N. Borisova, I. Kon, M. Lisina and others in their writings emphasize the fact that the function we are considering is most relevant in adolescence, which corresponds to the acmeological development of the personality. The following personality characteristics will be manifested in university students (Borisova E.V. 2006.):

- focus on actions;
- autonomy and self-regulation of behavior;
- creativity;
- responsibility for their actions and dids;
- effective interaction in society;
- the ability to reflection.

Ignoring this function in the process of development and formation of the personality of students leads to the fact that subsequently the desire to identify or reveal their potential fades; it also leads to apathy in relation to oneself, weak motivation, weak subject knowledge and skills; lack of initiative, preferring to act only under someone else's guidance.

Thus, we have characterized five basic functions through which not only the content, but also the structure of the acmeological development of the personality is manifested:

- the emotional-semantic component of the structure of psychological and acmeological development of a person is ensured by the function of self-understanding and self-development and is the basic acmeological position;
- the activity-value component is provided by the function of self-esteem and self-development, revealing the mechanisms of

acmeological formation and development of the learner's personality;

- behavioral and normative component is provided by the function of self-realization and self-affirmation of the student in vocational and educational activities. This component reveals the essence of the process of the formation of "acme", its productive aspect in the assimilation of the profession.

The above-mentioned functions, their characteristics and components of the acmeological development of the personality allow usadequately formulate the corresponding tasks for the development of personal "acme" among future specialists in the system of higher professional education.

Thus, understanding the content of the concept under consideration and its structure will allow us to determine the model of acmeological development of the personality of the future specialist, which will be reflected in obtaining the optimal result in its training.

The first criterion for the acmeological development of the personality of a future specialist is the development of the motivational sphere, i.e., students' motivation to achieve individual stages of personal growth. The study of professional motives makes it possible to consider a characteristic that guides the teacher's educational and professional activities and the development of his professional orientation. Professional motivation has a great influence not only on success in educational activities, but also on the formation of the student's professional competence. The effectiveness of the present educational activity of students, as well as the realization of their professional potential in the future, depends on the severity of professional motives. Along with the motivational component, the student develops a system of "acme" needs, which are a source of his activity and optimal development, including professional orientation.

A high level of acmeological personality development expresses the unity of interests in professional self-determination. The main content of its development is formed with an increase in the level of professional orientation. The choice of profession is justified when the activity of the person contributes to the relationship between the person and the activity, in which the creative and moral qualities of a student in higher education are successfully developed. A high level of professional orientation is one of the essential conditions for predicting personality development. The harmony of the key motive and the main content of the profession is a potential prerequisite for the search for "acme" in professional activities. The rest depends on the nature of the personality, the identity of personal qualities and the level of development of abilities. A system of social values lies at the core of the value orientations, perceivedas the individual value orientations.

Thus, when a student plans his future professional activity and himself in it, he proceeds from a certain hierarchy of values presented in his mind. He chooses precisely those values that are most closely linked to dominant needs. In the case when the value hierarchy is insufficiently formed, we are talking about inconsistency of value orientations: the student cannot make the choice of the most significant activity which he needs to focus his efforts on. A necessary criterion for the development of "acme" in this case is a clear formation of the value hierarchy of the individual and its consistency with his own value orientations and socio-cultural environment.

Developing in unity, the selected components have certain independence, autonomy, but the harmony of the personal and professional orientation depends on the level of development of each personality. Therefore, one of the practical tasks is to study the interconnections of structurally-substantive components of a professional orientation, which will allow us to determine the psychological and acmeological features of its development in connection with the possibility of optimization.

This conclusion served as the basis for questionnaire survey and forming a hierarchy of motivational-value orientations that are studied when developing a model of acmeological personality development using the example of students of the psychology department of the Institute of Pedagogy, Psychology and Inclusive Education of Humanities and Education Science Academy (branch) of V.I. Vernadsky Crimean Federal University in Yalta.

The acmeological development of the personality of a future specialist implies, first of all, the development of structurally meaningful components of his personality:

Cognitive component: reflects the totality of knowledge integrating ideas about the nature, laws of the processes of self-knowledge and self-development of a future specialist.

Activity component: the ability to implement the main areas of professional activity, formulate and solve professional problems, control, evaluate the results of your personal and professional activity, the ability to evaluate your professional level and the formation of an individual style of professional activity, due to self-organization and self-regulation.

At the motivational-value level, when planning his future professional activity, the student proceeds from a certain hierarchy of motives, which are the driving force for the development of professional competence. The values presented in his mind are also important, because by choosing precisely those motives and values that are most closely linked with dominant needs, he stimulates a future specialist to become more aware of the importance of owning self-processes and motivations for professional activity. In the case when a student does not express, for various reasons, the desire for professional self-improvement and self-development, or does not have the necessary skills, he needs psychological and pedagogical influence from the teachers of the department or psychological services of the educational institution of higher education.

In the process of acmeological development of the personality of students in higher education, goals and objectives, which are part of the structural components of the whole process of training a future specialist (Valeeva N. Sh. 2000), and indicate the specific content of each component of the model, come to the fore. So, the process of acmeological development of the personality of a student in a higher educational institution is subordinate to the following goals:

- assisting students with adaptation in the educational environment, the selection of landmarks in the context of educational and professional activities;

- promoting students' awareness of professional goals and motives;
- promoting the development of students' personality management skills and self-development in educational and professional activities;
- assisting in the development of its own acmeological program.

To achieve the goals you need to solve the following list of tasks:

- development of students' ability to self-actualization, self-government, self-regulation and self-development;
- adjustment of the system of values, needs, motives in the further professional and personal development;
- -development of an optimal model of personality development, professionally important qualities of students;
- assistance to students in the possibility of personal and professional development, promotion of independence in the search for ways of its optimal development.

The implementation of the goals and objectives of the acmeological development of the personality of the future specialist is ensured by the influence of internal factors, for example: the state of physical and mental health; motivational value sphere; cognitive sphere; activity component. And also, they depend on the influence of external factors, for example: information environment; socio-economic factors, etc. In turn, the realization of the goals and objectives of the optimal development of the personality of a future specialist is ensured by the joint efforts of all its subjects: teachers, students themselves, and the socio-cultural space.

In modern conditions and in this particular situation, subject-subject relations are preferable, suggesting the mutual activity and interaction of all participants in the educational process. Thus, the subjects of the process of acmeological personality development are both teachers and students themselves and that suggests their joint activity. The development process becomes optimal if it is determined by the subjective, creative forces of students, and it must pass through their internal sphere, mediates its activities and is implemented in it. The result of the effectiveness of the entire development process, as well as the development of structurally-meaningful components as a whole (motivational-value, cognitive, activity) is significantly affected by the activity of the socio-cultural environment. This is, first of all, the influence of family, the influence of friends and fellow students, faculty members, etc.

The main components of the acmeological model of the student's personality development are its algorithm and technology. Algorithm and technology occupy a central place and play an important role in the acmeological model.

The algorithm is a means of development and improvement is an important acmeological category developed by A. Derkach (Derkach A.A. and Sajko E.V. 2009).

So, the process of formation of an "acme" of the personality of a future specialist can be represented by the following algorithm:

- consciousness, life path goals in the context of educational and professional activities;
- clarification of the goals and objectives of the process of formation of "acme";
- decision and its planning, adopted on the basis of psychological and pedagogical support;
- -creation of optimal conditions for the development of the personality of a future specialist;
- -realization of the process of personality development of a future specialist;
- -control, self-assessment and adjustment of intermediate results of personality development of students in higher education.

Such algorithm becomes effective in the presence of effective technology. Technology is a combination of knowledge, information about methods and processes of their maintenance; set of techniques used in any business (Derkach A.A. and Sajko E.V. 2009).

Before proceeding with the description of the technology, it is necessary to formulate the most important requirements that should be taken into account when modeling the acmeological development of the personality of students in higher education.

The first is due to the fact that the whole complex of psychological phenomena, which determines the success of mastering knowledge, subjective characteristics of a person, potential opportunities and individual psychological characteristics of students, is not taken into account in the educational process, in which the main attention is paid only to the assimilation of theoretical knowledge, and not the formation of its basic professionally important qualities. At the same time, the dialectics of the development of psychological and acmeological science, the formation of a holistic view of the nature of man, the integration of scientific knowledge in the field of both theoretical and practical psychology, requires a change in the logic of the activities performed with the students, and in the standard algorithm. They must be aimed, first of all, at developing the ability for personal growth, personal and professional self-improvement and achieving "acme".

The second requirement is related to what special developmental and corrective measures must be included in the program of psychological and acmeological support for the development of the personality of a future specialist. Any program has clearly defined goals and objectives, involves a deeper approach to the development of the integrity of the individual and productivity increase in educational and professional activities and in life. All elements of the program, in particular, its individual and group options, are aimed both at developing personal growth, the formation of professional competence and professional development in general.

We believe that the fulfillment of these requirements is possible within the framework of a special technology that includes a combination of individual and group methods of work, taking into account the personal characteristics of students, as technologies of personal and professional self-improvement and self-development. Such a technology is a means of implementing the process of personality development, and simultaneously it provides a system of personal and professional self-development. It develops a holistic vision of a person, activates his values, needs, motives, interests, as well as internal creative resources of a person; combines conceptual knowledge and practical skills, skills with the ability to personal growth, as a result of which personal and professional development is achieved and, consequently, "acme".

The analysis of our study, as well as the above requirements, allowed us to identify models of acmeological personality development of students of higher educational institutions, which consist of five interrelated and complementary elements:

- adaptation;
- psycho diagnostic;
- professional and personal development;
- information orientation;
- education and correction.

1. Adaptation. This element is especially important for students and is an integral part of psychological support. Psychological support, in our opinion, should be carried out without fail regardless of the visible behavioral manifestations of students for the most successful inseparable inclusion in the educational process, which further contributes to the optimal development of a future specialist.
2. Psycho diagnostics. This element is necessary for optimal planning of the psychologist. For the implementation of an individual approach, diagnostics of the main psychological and acmeological characteristics of a person, as well as the general psychological state of students, is of great importance. This element allows you to find out the level of personality development and the formation of "acme" with a view to its further optimization and the possibility of correction.
3. Professionally-personal, developing element is aimed at personal and professional growth; it must mobilize the internal resources of the personality, adjust the basic psychological characteristics of

students, activate and develop professionally significant personality traits. These processes are basic and precede the successful development of the personality-professional orientation, contribute to self-actualization, self-regulation and self-development of the individual in achieving "acme".

4. Information and orientation. The presented element is necessary for the correct orientation in future personal and professional activities, as well as for the successful development of the personality in the learning process and revealing the prospects of the future profession, its features in order to form an adequate perception of it. Obtaining the full amount of information about future professional activities and obtaining a specialty helps the student to determine the goals and objectives of their activities, focused on the formation of professional competence.
5. Educational and correctional. This technology element includes the training of future specialists in the skills of self-realization, self-management, self-regulation, self-development, etc., the possibility of self-correction, as well as directly psychological and acmeological effects.

In this regard, our proposed model of acmeological development of the personality of students in higher education is a phased process:

Stage 1. It is mostly suitable for the first year of study, after a general introduction to the specialty. It involves acquaintance with students, establishing contact, conducting common simple test methods that can interest students, awaken their cognitive activity. This stage is based on the psycho diagnostic and information-orientation elements of the model. Its result is the orientation of students on future professional activities, the disclosure of its features.

Stage 2. In-depth psychological diagnostics in order to identify the level of development of all aspects of the personality, but the main attention should be paid to the study of structurally-substantive components that determine professional competence, since they are the most important for the optimal development and formation of the future professional and, in general, for the personality-professional acme. If it is necessary, the diagnosis should be carried out in several stages. The results of psycho diagnostics should become the basis for further work on the psychological and acmeological development of the personality of students.

Stage 3. The implementation of the program of psychological and acmeological development of the personality of students. Depending on the revealed level of personal and professional development, a group of students (or a student, if individual work is carried out) is included in the program, which can vary and be carried out using special methods and forms of work (trainings, practical exercises, exercises, various techniques focused on development of motivational-value structures of personality). The result of the third stage can be the development by students of their own program for the optimization of educational activities that clearly defines the setting of goals and objectives, as well as programming the students' actions, allowing them to be evaluated according to their own developed criteria, plan and predict a strategy for future activities to achieve the optimal level of acme development.

Stage 4. Generalization, control diagnostic procedures. Identification of the level of psychological and acmeological development of the personality of the future specialist, development of recommendations.

Each stage is a separate technology requiring detailed analysis. The implementation of the main stages of the psychological-acmeological development of the personality of a future specialist ensures its effectiveness, characterized by active successful educational activities and a clear formation of professional components. In this regard, it is of fundamental importance to optimize the system of psychological and acmeological development of the personality of a future specialist,developing the concept of criteria, indicators and levels reflected in the model.

A criterion acts as a sign on the basis of which an assessment, determination or classification of something takes place. The criterion expresses the essential changes in the object and is a means, a necessary assessment tool, but it is not the assessment itself. However, the choice of criterion is largely determined by the practical task of the study. In this case, it can be represented as a scientifically based model that expresses the essence of the object, the totality of knowledge of the results in which it is most expressed, or the sum of knowledge about the real achievements and capabilities of the object.

The criterion is a tool, a tool for assessing. The function of the criterion is the determination of the essential characteristics of the subject. The classification is based on a criterion.

When solving psychological problems, it is necessary to correctly determine the ratio of the concepts of a criterion and an indicator. An indicator and a criterion are particular and general, that is, any criterion contains indicators that qualitatively and quantitatively characterize it.

Acmeological criterion is the degree of professionalism, productivity of the subject of activity, as well as of personal and professional development. Acme criteria are integral, associated with fundamental manifestations of professionalism and more specific, reflecting the specifics of professional activity.

N. Kuzmina, studying the issues of professionalism of pedagogical activity, determined the measure of self-education and self-control, the measure of readiness for professional activity as the main criteria.

Currently, the essential criteria for acme are justified in acmeological studies, presented only in the potential human ability to achieve acme.

Acmeological indicators, in modern studies, are at the stage of completion of their formation, so it is customary to single out integral, specific and detailed indicators. The integral indicators of professional "acme" include:

- the effectiveness of professional activity;
- procedural characteristics of the activity;
- development of professional communication;
- maturity of the personality of a professional.

For specific acmeological indicators, one can determine the correlation of signs of mastery and professionalism of activity, by which it can be evaluated. The professionalism of an activity in its most general form can be characterized by the following indicators:

- a high level of cognitive abilities that ensure the stability of productivity and activity efficiency;
- high level of motivation;
- optimal intensity and intensity of labor;
- high accuracy and reliability;
- a high degree of self-organization;
- low mediation;
- creativity the possibility of the development of the subject of labor as a person;
- focus on achieving positive socially significant goals.

In the study, we proceeded from the fact that the indicators correspond to each criterion. The functional role of the criterion is in determining or not determining the essence of the formation of professional competence. Indicators, on the other hand, are a specific standard for assessing the development of the personality of students. In relation to this assessment, we identified groups of indicators that correspond to each criterion. Each criterion corresponds to a specific indicator and levels: high, sufficient, medium and low. So, guided by the analysis of scientific sources, we single out the substantive aspects of the criteria and indicators, presenting them in correlation, and create a common criteria-assessment base.

The cognitive criterion is correlated with indicators: self-knowledge and self-esteem, which make possible and deeper internal dialogue of the individual. The activity criterion is correlated with such indicators: professional skills, self-organization and self-regulation abilities. Motivational-value criterion is correlated with the following indicators: professional self-motivation and educational and professional values of the future specialist.

Thus, the general integration criterion of psychological and acmeological development of the personality of students in higher education is formulated as the optimality of the process, which reflects the essence of the phenomenon under study. Optimality means the best, in a sense, the most favorable. The optimal interaction between a person and his chosen professional activity is impossible without a sufficiently high level of professional orientation, since it is with the optimal development of the personality that the main content of this process is to increase its level:

- student readiness has a fixed relationship with the profession, interest in the presence of a pronounced nature of the cognitive criterion, which is variable. The practical side is aimed at the educational process, structured components of professional competency, etc.
- Installation on a profession, and more stable interests, the formation of inclinations, knowledge, abilities and skills of the practical side of the educational activity; formed structurally-substantive components of educational activity allow developing a sense of self-confidence, independence; there is a sense of responsibility.

The optimal development of professional competence is an indicator of a high level of acmeological development of the personality of students in higher education: the student shows a steady professional interest and an inclination to educational and professional activities and future specialties, shows particular enthusiasm for both the practical and theoretical side of the educational material;the process of their own educational and professional activities, self-assertion of the personality is taking place, the presence of a motive for professional mastery with clear convictions about the personal and social significance of their profession is noted.

REFERENCES

Andreev V.I. 2015. *Pedagogical heuristics for creative self-development of multidimensional thinking and wisdom: monograph.* Kazan': Centr innovacionnyh tekhnologij. 288 pp.

Baily K.D. 1982. *Methods of Social Research.* N.Y., London. 25 pp.

Bodalev A.A. 1998. *The pinnacle in adult development: Characteristics and conditions of achievement.* M.P. 20–21.

Borisova E.V. 2006. *The influence of the teacher's self-understanding on the productivity of professional and pedagogical communication:* dissertation thesis PhD in psychology. Astrahan'. Pp. 22.

Borytko N.M. 2005. *The system of professional education at the university: textbook.* allowancenauch. red. N.K. Sergeev. M.: APKiPRO. 120 pp.

Borytko N.M. and Mackajlova O.A. 2002. *The formation of the subjective position of the student in the humanitarian space of the lesson: Monograph.* Nauch. red. N. K. Sergeev. Volgograd: Izd-voVGIPKRO. 132 pp.

Derkach A.A. and Sajko E.V. 2009. "Self-realization as a structure-forming construct and process in ontogenesis (theoretical and methodological justification)"*Mir psihologii :Nauchno-metodicheskij zhurnal.* Red. D.I. Fel'dshtejn №2 (58) aprel'-iyun' 2009. P. 222-234.

Glinskij A.S. 2006. "Akmeology of the student and teacher". *Omskij nauchnyj vestnik.* №7 (43). P. 288–290.

Habermas Yu. 2001. *Moral consciousness and communicative action: translation from German.* SPb.:Nauka, 382 p.

Klimov E.A. 1995. *The image of the world in diverse professions.* M. MPSI. 127 pp.

Luk'yanova M.I. 2014. The formation of the acmeological position of the personality as a condition of professional and personal formation of the future specialist "*Sovremennyeproblemynaukiiobrazovaniya*". №5.

Maksimova V.N. 2002. *Introduction to acmeology of school education.* Spb. LOIRO. 156 pp.

Peshkova N.A. 2012. *Fundamentals of professional and personal self-development of a teacher.* Teaching aid.Tula: GOU DPO TO "IPK i PPRO TO", 264 pp.

Poletaeva N.M., Rodina E.A., Siyalova I.A., Lukina L.E. and others. 2014. *Internship of young teachers as a condition for the formation of professional maturity: Monograph.* SPb.: LGU im. A.S. Pushkina. 329 pp.

Puz'ko V.I. 2003. *Self-understanding and the crisis of personality: Monograph.* Mor. gos. un-tim. G. I. Nevel'skogo. Vladivostok : MGU. 322 p.

Rudakova O.A. 2019. "Acmeological development of the personality of the future psychologist as the basis of professional competence". *Problems of modern teacher education.* Ser.: Pedagogy and Psychology. Sat Articles: Yalta: RIO GPA, 2019. Issue. 63.1. P. 469–472.

Turgunbayeva B., Bekzhanova B., Uaidullakyzy E., Arkhabayeva D.A. 2013. Akmeological approach in professional training of the undergraduates in terms of postgraduate education. *Procedia. Social and Behavioral Sciences* 89 (2013). P. 544–548.

Valeeva N. Sh. 2000. *Scientific and pedagogical foundations for the training of managers of specialists for MP. Kazan.* gos. tekhnol. un-t. 208 pp.

In: Psychological Service ...
Editor: Svitlana V. Kucherenko
ISBN: 978-1-53618-160-9

Chapter 3

PSYCHOLOGICAL AND ACMEOLOGICAL DEVELOPMENT OF THE STUDENTS' PERSONALITY IN HIGHER SCHOOLS IN THE EDUCATIONAL ENVIRONMENT

Lyudmila V. Bura*[*]*, PhD
Psychology Department,
V. I. Vernadsky Crimean Federal University, Crimea, Russia

ABSTRACT

The chapter is devoted to the concept "student's adaptation." The adaptation process should be considered as a process aimed at achieving such a balance between the student and the educational environment in which the student can not only "adapt" and achieve "sustainability," but also is able to reveal his potential, to carry out positive environmental transformations. Socio-psychological adaptation can be decomposed into such components as socio-communicative, emotional-volitional, cognitive and psycho physiological component.

[*] Corresponding Author's Email: buraselivanova.l@mail.ru.

Keywords: acmeology, personality, student's adaptation, adaptation in a university, components of the adaptation process

INTRODUCTION

The educational environment is not just a certain space for activity, it is a multi-level interconnected system of conditions, elements and opportunities that contribute to the formation of the personality and its self-development. Accordingly, in the process of adaptation, not the individual's passive adaptation occurs, but, on the contrary, the student interacts actively with the environment in which changes occur in the cognitive, emotional-volitional, motivational and behavioral spheres of the personality. Factors or determinants (in fact, causes) affecting the integrity and success of a student's adaptation to study at a university are usually divided in the research psychological and pedagogical literature into objective, or external, and subjective, or internal. Objective factors include: gender, age, social environment, family relationships, specific conditions of study at a particular university (university location, material and technical base), pre-university training level, social and living conditions (change of residence, residence in a hostel), and others. Subjective factors include: individual psychological characteristics (memory, thinking, attention, willingness to study, level of intelligence, motivation, the necessary level of self-esteem and self-determination, formed communication skills, initiative, the availability of research abilities, etc.).

METHODS

Participants

After analyzing the scientific literature, we can identify the main criteria on the basis of which the researchers of this problem distinguish the components of university adaptation: student relations with teachers and the student group; adoption of standards of conduct adopted in a particular university; adoption of a new social role of a student; the effectiveness of social communication; the formation of new skills and habits; mastering the skills of independent work in educational and scientific activities; restructuring at a new level of all cognitive processes (perception, attention, memory, thinking); academic activity and academic performance; the student has the ability to self-development; level of intelligence, characteristics of learning and giftedness; the presence of a stable nature of reactions to events; positive emotional background; knowledge of the chosen profession; awareness of motives, goals and aspirations on the way to mastering the profession.

Considering the components of adaptation not as separate formations, but as the structure of the psychological construct "adaptation in an university" A. Smirnov and N. Zhivaev (Smirnov A. A. and Zhivaev N. G 2008) summarized such adaptation components as: social (reflects changes in the social sphere), didactic (reflects academic performance and processes associated with training) and professional (reflects the path to entering the professional environment).

While monitoring the adaptation of students at the university, I. Verchenko and K. Grineva (Verchenko I. A. and Grineva K. Yu. 2015) identified two components of adaptation: socio-psychological (reflects the personality's entry into the life of the learning environment, the adoption of its values and norms according to its interests and motives) and professional (adaptation to the chosen profession).

So, socio-psychological adaptation can be decomposed into such components as: socio-communicative, that reflect the ability to integrate into the learning environment through building communicative relationships with the environment; emotional-volitional that are responsible for a positive emotional attitude towards learning and selected prospects for professional development, manifesting in a low level of anxiety; cognitive component reflects academic performance and active participation in research projects; the psycho physiological component is realized in the absence of exacerbations of chronic diseases (Bura L. 2012).

Studying the process of adaptation of students of a branch university, L. Grechkina (Grechkina L. 2017) conducted a study of such structural interconnected components of adaptation as: social, didactic and professional. The author considers the student's personality, in particular, his individual qualities, inclinations, character and abilities as a unifying link that determines each of the components of adaptation. If we discard the indicators of low and high levels of adaptation, the average values for the components are very close and amounted to: social adaptation - 59%, didactic - 44%, professional - 41%. It should be noted that at the initial stage of the study, responding to a question about the motive for choosing a profession, 38% of respondents had a vague idea of their chosen professional activity. The main difficulties that arose in the learning process are related to congestion (26%), an uncomfortable class schedule (34%), lack or deficiency of free time (47%). All three types of problems can be attributed to the problem of rational planning and use of time. Statistically significant relationships between individual qualities and adaptation components were identified. As follows: a positive correlation between extraversion and the level of social adaptation and a high negative correlation between indicators of aggressiveness and didactic adaptation. No correlation of personal qualities with professional adaptation was found.

As part of the study of didactic adaptation of first-year students, E. Valteran and M. Krylova (Valteran E. and Krylova M. 2016) identified the necessary basic data for the diagnosis of the adaptation process of students in the first courses of the university. These are data on the characteristics of the student's motivational sphere, his personal attitude to the chosen field of study and the profession as a whole, school level, student satisfaction directly with the learning process, its quality, data on the difficulties that students face in the educational process, as in the classroom, and as a part of independent work.

The authors who studied the experience of adapting freshmen to the teaching on the basis of a pedagogical university, that developed a comprehensive program for the adaptation of first-year students, distinguish four components, such as:

- socio-psychological (the development of new types of behavior, self-organization and discipline and the adoption of the student's role in connection with entering the university's social environment, the student-teacher relationship system);
- professional (acquaintance with the requirements for a specialist of the chosen profession with subsequent familiarization with professional activity);
- didactic (reflects the student's ability to adapt to new forms of educational activity, volumes of knowledge and forms of knowledge control);
- physiological (the adoption of a new regime of "work-rest").

After conducting a sociological study, the authors identified factors that affect the components of the adaptation process (Bura L. 2012). Among the difficulties faced by students in terms of physiological adaptation, 42% note the problem of self-organization, 23% of students feel a lack of free time. The problems associated with didactic adaptation come down to indicators of the level of pre-university preparation (45% of students are inadequate), overload by the educational process (37%). Among the factors contributing to successful socio-psychological adaptation, 31% of students noted participation in cultural events. According to students (34%), indicators of professional adaptation were influenced by acquaintance with the university and listening to the course "Introduction to the specialty."

O. Arlashkina with co-authors (Arlashkina O. V., Naumova E. V. and Tevlyukova O. Yu. 2017) examined in detail, as part of the study of social adaptation of students, the adaptation for such components as academic, organizational, socio-psychological, psychophysiological and social. Conclusions, based on the materials of a sociological study, were drawn that both subjective and objective factors influence adaptation. At the same time, organizational, psychophysiological and social-everyday adaptation is more difficult. Physical and mental state of a student is accepted by the authors as the most significant subjective determinants for social adaptation.

A. Fedorinov (Fedorinov A. 2016) conditionally divided the freshmen's adaptability into three components: preparedness (basic knowledge and willingness to obtain specialized knowledge and skills according to the chosen specialty); social component (adaptation to the learning and living environment); material component (student's financial situation). The study sample was presented by graduates of large cities, rural schools, technical schools, freshmen with a time gap in education and foreign students. The analysis showed that of all students, the most prepared for the educational process at the university are graduates of secondary technical or special educational institutions, the least are graduates of rural schools.

The theory that graduates of rural schools compared with graduates of urban schools have lower adaptability indicators is confirmed by an experimental study by T. Dubovitskaya and A. Krylova (Dubovitskaya T. and Krylova A. 2010). According to the authors of the "Methodology for studying the adaptability of students in a university" in the first year of study, the most significant components are adaptation to the conditions of educational activity and adaptation to the study group. The conditions of educational activity, in particular, include the forms of teaching at the university, knowledge control, the mode of study and rest. Adaptation to a study group means communication between fellow students. In essence, these concepts are very similar to social and didactic adaptation. As for professional adaptation (the development of professional skills), the authors attribute it to the period of senior courses and do not take it into account in this study.

An investigation, carried out to identify the degree of adaptation of students in connection with changes in living conditions when entering a university, identified a number of problems that cause difficulties in the process of adaptation (Grechkina L. 2017). Students identified the components that influenced the adaptation process. The percentage of the survey of the total number of respondents was: didactic (related to the training mode and academic load) – 56.3%; social welfare (in particular, associated with living in a dormitory or rented housing) – 66.7%; psychological (related to getting used to independent life, living in a new city) – 45.3%; communicative (in relations with teachers and fellow students) – 26.7%.

M. Babushkina and E. Feskova (Babushkina M. and Feskova E. 2012) identified four interconnected and interdependent adaptation substructures in their study of the features of the adaptation process: social, didactic, psychological and physical. The aim of the experiment, carried out with first-year students of the university, was to determine the level of formation of these types of adaptation.

According to the results of the study, it can be argued that the physical adaptation to the learning process was most favorable among respondents (38%), psychological and social adaptation were at about the same level (24% and 22%, respectively), the lowest level was recorded relative to didactic adaptation – 16%. Based on the results obtained, it can be concluded that, as in the previously mentioned studies, the most difficult thing for a student in the first months is to adapt to everything that is directly related to the educational process. It is much easier to build relationships with classmates and the teaching staff.

Similar results with respect to the social component were obtained in an empirical study by N. Golubeva. and A. Golovanova (Golubeva N. and Golovanova A. 2014), the purpose of whom was to detect statistically significant relationships between individual personality characteristics and adaptation components. A high level of social adaptation is associated with the extraversion of the personality. A person with such qualities as impulsiveness, sociability, initiative, social openness, tolerance is more successful in the process of social adaptation. However, in this study, regulatory flexibility became the most significant and rather universal adaptation factor. According to this personality trait, the maximum number of connections with adaptation parameters is observed. In other words, the higher the individual's ability to adequately assess the prevailing conditions and results of activities, the higher the level of emotional comfort and poise.

Such a personal quality as initiative, and its importance in the process of adaptation, is given special attention in one of the studies on the conditions for successful adaptation of students to educational loads. The authors, agreeing with some researchers, believe that a competent specialist is a product of personal self-development (Dubovitskaya T. and Krylova A. 2010). Self-development can be achieved by shifting the emphasis in the learning process from teacher activity to student activity, which is manifested by initiative and responsibility. Initiative is considered as an integrative quality, combining structural elements. The connecting link in the chain of components is the need-motivating element, while motivation is created on the basis of needs. In turn, the emotional-volitional component ensures the realization of the motive by regulating behavior and performing purposeful activities. Communicative-active component is manifested in the willingness to realize their capabilities.

According to N. Fomina and I. Bakova (Fomina N. A. and Bakova I. V. 2010), problems in adaptation and personal development of students may arise due to certain difficulties in communication, since communication is an important property of the personality and corrector of the emotional-volitional sphere, representing a basis for building interpersonal relationships. This hypothesis is confirmed by an experimental study. The authors found that socio-psychological adaptation in communicative students proceeds differently than in non-communicative students. The successful adaptation of non-communicative students is affected by such personal and behavioral components as low self-esteem, statement, tendency to obey, hostile attitude towards others, low level of volitional self-regulation and negative emotional background.

According to I. Labyntseva (Labyntseva I. 2010), the successful adaptation of a student in general depends on his motivation and conscious choice of future professional activity. She carried out an empirical study, the results of which prove this hypothesis. There is a direct correlation of personal choice and successful student adaptability at the initial stage of training. The studied sample of students was divided into two groups. One group included students (39% of respondents) who showed awareness when choosing a profession, which is expressed in the confidence that the chosen specialty corresponds to personal goals and abilities and the intention to work in the chosen specialty. The other group included students who chose the appropriate profession, who showed insecurity or fears of an erroneous choice, lack of intentions to perform professional activities in their specialty (28% of respondents).

The generalized experimental results indicate that in the first group the level of educational activity, indicators of motivation, satisfaction with the educational process are much higher than in the second one. Students of the first group differ in terms of emotional comfort, acceptance of the student's role and harmonious relationships with the environment. Accordingly, students of the first group are more successful in the adaptation process than students of the second group.

In the work of S. Kusakina (Kusakina S. 2008) the problem of motivation for studying at a university is considered as one of the components of readiness for learning. In turn, readiness is seen as the main criterion for academic performance. Thus, the author identified the following components of readiness for learning: motivation (immediate desire to study, fulfill duties that correspond to the status of a student and the goals of entering a university); intellectual development (availability of necessary basic knowledge); volitional component (self-organization, activity in the process of cognition, perseverance); motor-organizational component (speed of writing and reading, the ability to switch attention quickly, the skills of working with text); professional component (awareness of the choice of a future profession and a desire to master it).

The student's psychological readiness for the educational process is given special attention, since the coordination of personal qualities and educational activities ensures the effective development of activities that are important for gaining knowledge and skills, such as cognitive, research, self-development and self-education. In particular, in the works by F. Gemeshliev and N. Lyz (Gemeshliev F. and Lyz N. 2011) a model that reflects the relationship between the components of preparedness and the proper areas of personality has been developed. So, motivation, as one of the components, is based on the awareness of their goals, planned achievements, life guidelines, prospective development prospects, and self-realization. In other words, motivation is interconnected with the value-semantic sphere of a person. The regulatory component correlates with the emotional-volitional sphere, which is implemented in the rational use of time, overcoming difficulties, concentration, mobilization of one's own forces, control and correction of activity. The cognitive sphere of the personality (attention, memory, thinking, etc.) acts as the basis for the intellectual component (the ability to understand, assimilate and transform the knowledge gained). The acquired knowledge and skills are the basis for mastering the chosen profession (the "knowledge-operational" component), representing a part of the student's cumulative experience, and are related to the sphere of the individual's experience.

The importance of the motivational component and readiness for the learning process were investigated by G. Sholokhova. and I. Chikova (Sholokhova G. and Chikova I. 2014) in determining the psychological and pedagogical features of adaptation to learning. Among the respondents, out of the total number of which 33.3% chose the appropriate university during the last year of schooling, the percentage ratio for the factors of university choice was: interest in the profession (40.1%); choice by analogy with peers (23.2%), desire to get a diploma (16.7%), parents' choice (20%). The greatest difficulties that students encountered in the first year of study are directly related to the learning process (60% of respondents). The main reason for the occurrence of difficulties of this nature is insufficient basic training, in particular, 40% experience a lack of knowledge in some disciplines, and 20% of the entire sample have the same problem in all subjects. According to the results of the investigation, the majority of students noted the presence of fatigue, a decrease in motivation for the educational process and profession (63.3%).

The influence of motivation on the successful adaptation process is confirmed in the work of O. Balykina and N. Seregina (Balykina O. and Seregina N. 2016). The diagnostic result for two generalized stable motives of the personality such as the desire for success and the avoidance of failure, were the following data. Before taking a course of motivational trainings, motivation to avoid failure prevailed among students (September

– 60.33%), and after the course motivation for success prevailed (December – 54.76%).

Researchers Thomas Hamilton Bailey and Lisa J. Phillips (Bailey T. H. and Phillips L. J. 2016) assessed the degree of motivation influence on successful adaptation to learning and its relationship with subjective well-being. The study is based on the theory of self-determination, according to which the authors divide motivation into internal (learning from the interest of acquiring new knowledge and skills for the purpose of self-development) and external (motives of duty, responsibility, etc.). By initiating educational activities for their own sake and their internal interests, in the process of searching for new opportunities and implementing new behavioral styles, students, driven by internal motivation, are distinguished by a higher level of cognitive and social development. According to the results of the study, the hypothesis that students, driven by intrinsic motivation, are more successful in social, emotional, academic adaptation and have a higher level of psychological health was confirmed.

The relationship of individual qualities and the successful adaptation of first-year students were studied by A. Shklyarova (Shklyarova A. 2017). Thus, according to the results of the study, emotional stability and extroversion are defined as individual characteristics that affect the success of the adaptation process. There is a strong direct connection between these qualities and adaptation. This conclusion is made on the basis of statistically significant direct relationships between extraversion and the acceptance of others; emotional stability and self-acceptance, acceptance of others, emotional comfort, internality, desire for dominance. It should also be noted that if extroversion seems to be an innate quality of the individual, then emotional stability can be corrected.

The same indicators of socio-psychological adaptation were studied by S. Khonsky (Khonsky S. 2017) with a detailed research of student's gender and profile. So, according to the results of the study, there are some gender differences. An analysis of the emotional state and communicative abilities of students of a technical university was carried out by L. Yasyukova and O. Piskun (Yasyukova L. and Piskun O. 2009). The average values of the studied parameters allowed the authors to determine the factors that impede the adaptation process. All maladaptive students have a low level of tolerance, which (according to the correlation analysis) has a particularly significant relationship with the emotional state. Such students are characterized by prejudice, intolerance, aggressiveness, low level of control of their emotions, irritability. Among young men, a depressed emotional state is mainly found in emotionally inactive persons, who is in need of support and is skeptical by nature. In female students, maladaptation is associated with such personal qualities as shyness, conservatism. All of the above mentioned qualities significantly affect the communication opportunities and social contacts in a multicultural environment, thereby complicating the process of adaptation.

The influence of intelligence features on the students' adaptation process is determined in another study of the same authors. In particular, according to the results of the study, the authors concluded that the logical component of conceptual thinking is influenced by successful adaptation to learning, since at a low level of its development it becomes impossible to understand the essence of the material being studied and to form adequate scientific ideas.

A wide variety of criteria for assessing the success of adaptation similar to existing definitions of the term "adaptation" are proposed in the scientific literature. In particular, V. Gribov (Gribov V. 1999) describes the following criteria:

- students' satisfaction with studying at a university, which is reflected in conditions of interpersonal relations, justified ideas about the chosen profession;
- the effectiveness of the learning process (academic performance);
- activity manifested not only in the educational, but also in the public life of the university;
- self-satisfaction, which is reflected in the level of anxiety, adequate self-esteem, potential realization, etc.
- Adaptation criteria, according to P. Kuznetsov (Kuznetsov P. 1991) are as follows:

- assimilation of knowledge, fulfillment of social roles, social status occupied by the individual in the system of interpersonal relations;
- relationships with others, determining the development of the individual at this stage;
- the level of development of self-identity of the person and the degree of manifestation of the subject-active principle, both in relation to his environment, and in relation to himself, as an object and subject.

O. Zotova and I. Kryazheva (Zotova O. and Kryazheva I. 1988) consider the criteria for socio-psychological adaptation, dividing them into subjective and objective. Subjective ones include satisfaction with oneself and one's life, emotional and physical comfort. Objective criteria are productivity, real situation in the team, the indicators of which are academic performance and overall health.

After analyzing the results of modern research on the adaptation of first-year students, it can be concluded that subjective and objective factors, as well as criteria for evaluating the effectiveness of the process, should be considered in the context of adaptation conditions. Moreover, it is indisputable that the successful adaptation of students is necessary and prerequisite for further professional and personal growth. The adaptation process should be considered as a process aimed at achieving such a balance between the student and the educational environment in which the student can not only "adapt" and achieve "sustainability," but also is able to reveal his potential, to carry out positive environmental transformations.

References

Arlashkina O. V., Naumova E. V. and Tevlyukova O. Yu. "Social adaptation of first-year students at the university (based on research)" *Teoriya i praktika obshchestvennogo razvitiya*. 2017. № 11. P 54–58.

Babushkina M. A. and Fes'kova E. V. "Peculiarities of the adaptation of students in high school." *Molodyozh' i nauka: Sbornik materialov VIII*

Vserossijskoj nauchno-tekhnicheskoj konferencii studentov, aspirantov i molodyh uchyonyh, posvyashchennoj 155-letiyu so dnya rozhdeniya K. E. Ciolkovskogo [Elektronnyj resurs]. Krasnoyarsk: Sibirskij federal'nyj un-t, 2012.

Bailey T. H. and Phillips L. J. The influence of motivation and adaptation on students' subjective well-being, meaning in life and academic performance. *High Educ Res Dev*. 2016. Vol. 35. Pp. 201–216.

Balykina, O. S. *Motivational training as a means of adapting students to study at a university*/O. S. Balykina, N. V. Seregina//Vestnik Bryanskogo gosudarstvennogo universiteta. 2016. №3. Pp. 257–262.

Bura L. V. "Description of external and internal factors affecting the process of adaptation of students in a new social development situation" *Innovacionnye tekhnologii v obrazovanii: materialy VIII Mezhdunarodnoj nauchno-prakticheskoj konferencii "Innovacionnye tekhnologii v obrazovanii*": sbornik statej. Yalta: RVUZ KGU, 2012. Pp. 27–28.

Dubovickaya T. D. and Krylova A. V. "Methodology for studying the adaptability of students at a university" *Psihologo-pedagogicheskie issledovaniya*. 2010. № 2. Pp. 1–7.

Fedorinov A. V. "Adaptaciya pervokursnikov k obucheniyu v Gosudarstvennom universitete po zemleustrojstvu i vozmozhnosti ee sovershenstvovaniya [*Adaptation of freshmen to study at the State University for land management and the possibility of its improvement*]: sbornik statej i tezisov po itogam Kruglogo stola, posvyashchennogo problemam adaptacii studentov-pervokursnikov"; pod redakciej N. I. Ivanova, M. V. Borisovoj, V. V. Men'shih, N. A. Mihalevoj. M. GUZ, 2016. Pp. 90–96.

Fomina N. A. and Bakova I. V. A comparative analysis of the features of socio-psychological adaptation of students with different structural organization of sociability. *Izvestiya Samarskogo nauchnogo centra RAN*. 2010. № 3–2. Pp. 447–450.

Gemeshliev F. K and Lyz' N. A. "A model of students' psychological readiness for mastering vocational training programs" *Izvestiya*

Yuzhnogo federal'nogo universiteta. Tekhnicheskie nauki. 2011. № 10 (123). Pp. 162–168.

Golubeva N. M. and Golovanova A. A. "Factors of students' adaptation to the educational environment of the university" *Izvestiya Saratovskogo universiteta. Novaya. seriya. Akmeologiya obrazovaniya. Psihologiya razvitiya.* 2014. T. 3. № 2 (10). Pp. 125–130.

Grechkina L. Yu. "Studying the adaptation process of university students" *Vestnik Buryatskogo gosudarstvennogo universiteta. Pedagogika*. Ulan-Ude: Izd-vo Buryat. gos. un-ta. 2017. № 1. Pp. 3–9.

Gribov V. N. *Adaptation of the youth of a small Siberian city to the conditions of study at the university*: dissertation thesis PhD in pedagogy. Tyumen', 1999. 23 pp.

Honskij S. I. *Differences in the characteristics of socio-psychological adaptation of students at the initial stage of study at a university*. Sofiya. 2017. № 1. Pp. 27–32.

Kusakina, S. N. "Motivation for entering a university for high school students and students." *Psihologicheskaya nauka i obrazovanie*. 2008. № 1. Pp. 58–66.

Kuznecov P. S. *Adaptation as a function of personality development*. Saratov: Izd-vo Saratovskogo universiteta, 1991. 70 pp.

Labynceva, I. S. Adaptation of teaching students at the university with different subjective reasons for choosing a profession. Izvestiya YuFU. *Tekhnicheskie nauki*. 2010. № 10 (111). Pp. 198–203.

Shklyarova A. A. "The relationship of personal characteristics and the adaptation of first-year students to higher education" *Nauchno-metodicheskij elektronnyj zhurnal "Koncept"*. 2017. T. 12. Pp. 120–124.

Sholohova G. I. and Chikova I. V. Adaptation of freshmen to the conditions of study at the university and its psychological and pedagogical features. *Zhurnal "Vestnik Orenburgskogo gosudarstvennogo universiteta*." 2014. №3 (164). Pp. 103–107.

Smirnov A. A. and Zhivaev N. G. *The psychology of university adaptation: teaching aid.* Yarosl. gos. un-t im. P. G. Demidova. Yarovlavl': YarGU, 2009. 115 pp.

Val'teran, E. V. and Krylova M. A. *"Adaptaciya pervokursnikov k vuzovskoj srede v sisteme studencheskogo samoupravleniya*" [*"Theoretical foundations of the study of didactic adaptation of students"*]: sbornik statej i tezisov po itogam Kruglogo stola, posvyashchennogo problemam adaptacii studentov-pervokursnikov; pod redakciej N. I. Ivanova, M. V. Borisovoj, V. V. Men'shih, N. A. Mihalevoj. M.: GUZ, 2016. Pp. 9–15.

Verchenko I. A. and Grineva K. Yu. "Assessment of the success of adaptation of first-year students to the conditions of the university." *Vestnik Chelyabinskogo gosudarstvennogo pedagogicheskogo universiteta*. 2015. № 9. Pp. 131–135.

Yasyukova L. A. and Piskun O. E. Gender features of students' adaptation of studing at a technical university. *Zdorov'e – osnova chelovecheskogo potenciala: problemy i puti ih resheniya*. 2009. № 1. Pp. 260–262.

Zotova O. I. and Kryazheva I. K. Some aspects of the socio-psychological adaptation of personality. *M. Medicina*, 1988. 256 pp.

In: Psychological Service … ISBN: 978-1-53618-160-9
Editor: Svitlana V. Kucherenko

Chapter 4

RESEARCH OF THE UNIVERSITY PSYCHOLOGICAL SERVICE: CAREER ANCHORS OF UNDERGRADUATES AND STUDENTS IN THE MASTER'S PROGRAMME IN MAJOR IN THE CONDITIONS OF THE HIGHER EDUCATION

***Svitlana V. Kucherenko*[*,1], PhD**
***and Tatiana P. Pavliuk*[2], PhD**
[1]Psychology Department,
V.I. Vernadsky Crimean Federal University,
Yalta, Crimea, Russia
[2]Department of Humanities,
V.I. Vernadsky Crimean Federal University,
Armiansk, Crimea, Russia

[*]Corresponding Author's Email: kusvitlana@gmail.com.

Abstract

This Chapter discusses the results of a study of career attitudes of University students and master's degree students of Academy of Humanities of V.I. Vernadsky Crimean Federal University. It reveals the possibilities of using the directed associative test and flow of associations in the study of students' career preferences. The study involved 163 people from the bachelor's program of the specialty "Practical psychology" (n = 31), master's programs (n = 132) of the specialty "Computer Science. Mathematics" (n = 17), "Psychology" (n = 13), "Design" (n = 9), "Finance" (n = 11), "Management" (n = 7), "Management of higher education" (n = 25), "Inclusive education" (n = 9), "History" (n = 2), "Music" (n = 3), and "Philology" (n = 36). The directed associative test in combination with the questionnaire "career anchors" by E. Shane opens up opportunities for learning the unique inner world of each individual, including in the field of career attitudes and expectations.

As a result of an empirical study, a lower degree of orientation to the stability of the place of residence was revealed with a high orientation to the stability of the work place of Crimean students. This may indicate that students and undergraduates of the Pedagogy and Humanities Academy are less likely to seek competence in their careers (Professional competence, Management and Entrepreneurship), while there is an emotional oversupply about the career anchors of needs (Autonomy, Security - the stability of the place of residence and Pure challenge), thus we can talk about an intrapersonal conflict.

Keywords: career anchors, career preferences, directed associative test, directed flow of associations

Introduction

In today's dynamic and unstable socio-economic situation, the tasks associated with the building and developing a career become very relevant for psychology, thanks to which a person has the possibility to realize his abilities, opportunities and fulfil needs. Psychological researches in this area are quite diverse (Volkova 2018; 2016). Also the features of career anchors of students at the final stage of University education are studied

(Lozhechkina, Bakunova, Tkachenko 2017), but there wasn't paid attention to the process of their development and transformation.

As during the period of study at the University there is a formation of career anchors, this is reflected in the specifics of needs, values, career goals and developing career plans that determine the success of career and professional development in general. The acquisition of specific ideas of professional and personal future, requirements imposed on representatives of a particular profession is exactly characterized for the stage of late youth.

The specificity of career settings of representatives of various professional orientations was studied by Lozhechkina A. D. (Lozhechkina A. D. 2017), Bakunova I. V. and Tkachenko A. V. (Bakunova, Tkachenko 2017). An investigation of career anchors of Iranian software engineers consisting of needs, values and competencies was performed by Alavi S. B., Moteabbed S. (Alavi, S. B., Moteabbed, S., Arasti, M. R. 2012). Authors describe the composition of career anchors as follows (Table 1).

From the Table 1, you can see that all career anchors fall into three groups: needs, values, and competencies. Entrepreneurship can represent both value and competence, so we have assigned this career anchor to both groups.

METHODS

Directed Associative Test

Associative experiment is used in psychology as a projective method of diagnostics of motivational sphere of personality (Large psychological dictionary 2007, 41–42). A free associative experiment was proposed by C. G. Jung, M. Wertheimer and D. Klein. The respondent is asked to respond to a certain stimulus (word) with any word that comes to his mind for a certain time (10–15 min.). The type of emerging associations, the frequency of similar and repeated associations, the value of time periods (pauses) between the responses of the subject, behavioral and physiological reactions are recorded. The method of free and directed associations is used in psycholinguistics to study the psychosemantics of the word (Ivanova, N. A. 2013) and in sociology to study various socio-psychological phenomena with the consideration of the "associative field" and the "core of the associative field" of the person (Golenkova, L. A., Chernyaeva, V. V. 2013).

Table 1. Composition of career anchors (Alavi, S. B., Moteabbed, S., Arasti, M. R. 2012)

Needs	Values	Competencies
Autonomy	Sense of service/ dedication	Professional competence
Security (the stability of the place of residence/ the place of work)	Life style integration	Management
Pure challenge	Entrepreneurship	Entrepreneurship

The resulting stream of associations is subjected to categorical and content analysis. Let us consider an example of the analysis of the directed chain flow of associations by the method of C. G. Jung on the stimulus (word) "career":

"Knowledge, movement, light, speed, exchange, study, communication, catalyst, board, step, forward, reaction, space, calm, melting, cold, speed, dispersion, communication, accuracy, drop, letter, guide, coffee, energy, movement, fire, flame, grass, sign, curve, smirk, communication, person, attachment, shackles, cargo, responsibility, boredom, slander, measles, bloom, rumble, dawn, wasp, noise, bumblebee, poison, bush, shore, surf, silence, womb, decision, plan, list, purpose, union".

The associations are grouped into the following semantic units:

1. Pedagogy – knowledge, study, board, guide, plan (5 words).
2. Psychology – communication, exchange, calmness, communication, person, attachment, responsibility, boredom, decision, goal (10 words).

3. Physics – motion, light, speed, precision, sign, curve, dispersion, energy, melting, cold, cargo, space (12 words).
4. Chemistry – catalyst, drop, fire, flame (4 words).
5. Medicine – measles, reaction, womb (3 words).
6. Nature – bush, shore, surf, bloom, dawn, wasp, bumblebee, grass (8 words).
7. Concrete objects and phenomena – smirk, slander, rumble, list, coffee (5 words).

Thus, the hierarchy of semantic units of this directed flow of associations is as follows: physical concepts are in the first place, psychological – on the second and describing nature – on the third. It can be concluded that the respondent's picture of the world is mainly mechanistic; psychology and nature are also relevant. The final word is union, that is, career is understood as a way of integrating with other people and social members.

This stream of associations was received in 10 minutes; pauses were few after the words "speed" and "communication"; the author was a student in the master's programme in major of "V.I. Vernadsky Crimean Federal University" of psychology department. You can make a coherent text with these words, which can be subsequently analyzed by the method of narrative analysis.

Shane's Career Anchor Questionnaire

Let us compare the results with the marking of career anchors according to E. Shane. Professional competence – 4 points, management – 5 points, autonomy – 8 points, stability of residence – 2 points, stability of work – 3 points, sense of service – 7 points, pure challenge – 7 points, life style integration – 8 points, entrepreneurship – 9 points. Thus, our respondent is dominated by career orientations of entrepreneurship, life style integration and autonomy.

The overwhelming majority of words of the directed stream of associations concerned physical phenomena and names of the nature that testifies to mechanistic understanding of autonomy as separate abstraction, instead of real quite concrete independence. Among psychological terms there are mainly names of communicative processes and qualities that characterize connectivity and attachment rather than autonomy. The result is an intrapersonal conflict between the desire to belong to other people and identify oneself with them and autonomy, which is a prerequisite for entrepreneurship. These associations are more consistent with the career attitude of "service" than "autonomy", "life style integration" or "entrepreneurship".

As can be seen from Table 2, this individual profile of career anchors is dominated by values, namely, sense of service and life style integration. The source of internal psychological tension of this author of the directed flow of associations is presumably the *contradiction between the desire for autonomy* according to the results of the questionnaire "Career anchors" by E. Shane and the *lack of faith in their own abilities to achieve independence* (colloquial words *smirk, slander, rumble, list*, which have a negative emotional coloring). Thus, the direction of corrective action for this respondent will be the study of their own desire for autonomy as well as awareness and clarification of this career anchor.

Let's consider another directed stream of associations to the "career" stimulus. It concludes: psychology, music, art, learning, development, *culture*, exercise, sport, interaction, association, *benefit*, purpose, stimulus, action, conclusion, response, light, darkness, colors, sense, meaning, significance, symbol, image, silhouette, nature, travel, *culture*, myths, reality, relationship, metaphor, allegory, parable, information, painting, history, project, presentation, discovery, explanation, freedom, expression, versatility, *benefit*, blue, green, yellow, serenity, society, tranquility, loneliness, thoughts, actions, reactions, hours, infinity, interest, constructions, history, facts, logic, aphorism, feelings, morality, emptiness. According to the specified the following categories of associations can be distinguished: psychology (18 words), art (14 words), philosophy (16 words), pedagogy (11 words), physics (10 words), freedom (5 words), sports and history (2 words each).

Table 2. Categorical connections between career attitudes and semantic units of the chain flow of associations on the stimulus "career" of the first-year student in the master's program in major of the specialty "Psychology"

Professional competence	Management	Autonomy	The stability of the place of residence	The stability of the place of work	Sense of service/ dedication	Pure challenge	Life style integration	Entrepreneurship
4 points	5 points	8 points	2 points	3 points	7 points	7 points	8 points	9 points
5 words		5 words		3 words	10 words	4 words	8 words	12 words
learning		concrete objects		medicine	psychology	chemistry	nature	physics

Needs: 5 + 0 + 3 + 4 = **12 words, Values:** 10 + 8 + 12 = **30 words** and **Competencies:** 5 + 0 + 12 = **17 words**.

Table 3. Categorical relations between career attitudes and semantic units of the chain flow of associations on the stimulus "career" of the second-year undergraduate student of the specialty "Psychology"

Professional competence	Management	Autonomy	The stability of the place of residence	The stability of the place of work	Sense of service/ dedication	Pure challenge	Life style integration	Entrepreneurship
7 points	7 points	5 points	5 points	5 points	8 points	4 points	4 points	4 points
16 words	11 words	14 words	2 words		18 words	2 words	10 words	5 words
Philosophy	Pedagogy	Art	History		Psychology	sport	physics	freedom

Needs: 14 + 2 + 0 + 2 = **18 words, Values:** 18 + 10 + 5 = **33 words** and **Competencies:** 16 + 11 + 5 = **32 words**.

As can be seen from Table 3, in comprehension of this respondent, the prevailing career anchor "service" corresponds to the category of psychology with the semantically loaded word "benefit"; professional competence corresponds to the category of philosophy ("culture", "logic"); "management" – the category of pedagogy, "autonomy" – art; "stability of residence" – history; "life style integration" – physics ("light" and "darkness"); "entrepreneurship" – freedom. The source of intrapersonal conflict is the contradiction between the frequency of occurrence of words of the category "art" and the lack of expression of the corresponding career attitude "autonomy", that is, unconsciously the autonomy is important for the author, but consciously he pushes this career attitude to the background. The direction of the corrective impact for this respondent will also be the work on the awareness of their own desire for autonomy.

The stream of associations ends with the word "emptiness", which has been categorized as "physics" and correlated with the career anchor of "integrating lifestyles". That is, the author perceives career in the context of combination (alternation) with other spheres of life.

Let's consider the flow of associations on the stimulus "career" of the third-year student of the specialty "Psychology". They are: mountain, peak, maximum, success, prosperity, multi-employment, security, wealth, money, currency, shopping, car, travel, island, vacation, sea, depth, meaning, life, family, wealth, health, happiness, children, smile, joy, well-being, house, brick, castle, Princess, beauty, fame, success, reward, recognition, development, movement, growth, achievement, business, responsibility, honesty, justice, honesty, nobility, love, man, support, strength, courage, protection, peace, peace, understanding, sensitivity, kindness, openness, freedom, breath, ease, carefree, calm, peace, stability, power, status, head, head, leader, leader, rod, confidence, group, subordinates, employees, work, fruitfulness, result, goal, center, idea, explosion, grandiosity, utility, significance, result, success, top, power, strength, firmness, power, rigidity, order, manner, democracy, friendship, goodwill, smile, sincerity, openness, honesty, justice, rod, pillar, position, confidence, self-control, self-regulation, management, leadership, power, openness, honesty.

The following categories of associations can be distinguished: acme ("top", "growth", "success") – 14 words, power – 21 words, morality ("core", "honesty") – 13 words, self-regulation and self-esteem ("calmness", "peace", "confidence") – 17 words, result – 8 words, family and relationships – 7 words, wealth – 16 words, recognition ("business", "fame") – 6 words, physics and abstract concepts – 4 words.

As can be seen from Table 4, this third-year student of the specialty "Psychology" understands professional competence as the achievement of peaks in life, management – as a reliance on the moral qualities of the individual ("core", "honesty"), autonomy – as the ability to self-regulation ("calm", "peace", "confidence"). **Needs:** 43 words, **Values:** 36 words and **Competencies:** 48 words. Entrepreneurship is perceived by the author as the realization of their own power ambitions, career anchor "pure challenge" corresponds to the desire for wealth and material security, contradictory attitude to which is a source of intrapersonal conflict. That is, the student strives for material security, but is not ready for competition, difficulties and risks associated with it.

Let's review the average values according the method of "Career anchors" in groups of master's degree students and undergraduates of the second and third years (Table 5).

As can be seen from Table 5, of all the studied groups of undergraduates and master's degree students of Academy of humanities and pedagogy, the highest values of career anchors are observed in the group of extramural master's degree students, the lowest – in intramural students of the bachelor's degree. However, compared to the students of the Vladivostok state University of Economics and service, they have much less expressed career anchors such as management (7.59 compared to 6.28 and 6.14), autonomy (7.19 compared to 7.13 for masters and 6.35 for bachelors) and stability of residence (6.2 compared to 4.74 and 4.79). Differences in the manifestation of career anchor "management" can be explained by the specifics of economic specialties of Vladivostok University, since students of Humanities in Academy of humanities and pedagogy are less likely to seek to manage other people. The differences in "autonomy" are within the standard deviation, so they are not significant.

However, the less expressed orientation to the stability of the place of residence with a high orientation to the stability of the place of work of Crimean students indicates less attachment to the place of living and the desire to leave their hometown in order to build a career in the chosen direction. It is advisable to check these empirical results on a larger sample of other universities in the Crimea in order to exclude situational influence and regional aspect (Yalta city).

Peculiar properties of career anchors of students of pedagogical specialties of the first and fifth courses were described in the works of O. P. Ternovskaya (Ternovskaya 2006). The typical career anchor for the majority of graduate students of pedagogical University appeared to be “stability of work”; not typical – anchors “pure challenge” and “autonomy”, that suggest competition, freedom from restrictions and regulations, which are quite consistent with the future work of the teacher, associated with cooperation and work in a stable organization. At the same time, the most significant orientation for students of specialties of Humanities is “sense of service”, for students of natural specialties – “stability of work”, for students of mathematical specialties “entrepreneurship”. Significant differences between the initial and final course were found in relation to career anchors of “professional competence” and “entrepreneurship”: “the first-year students’ choice of competence was more represented, while orientation to “entrepreneurship” became more significant for the graduates.

Self-Presentation Strategies Questionnaire

Interpersonal self-presentation has been studied extensively by psychologists and sociologists. This concept was developed by Goffman (1959) who described how people negotiate and validate their identities in face-to-face communication and introduced “frames” within which to evaluate the meaning of interpersonal encounters (Ahmed A. 2014).

Table 4. Categorical relations between career attitudes and semantic units of the chain flow of associations on the stimulus "career" of the third-year student of the specialty "Psychology"

Professional competence	**Management**	**Autonomy**	**The stability of the place of residence**	**The stability of the place of work**	**Sense of service/ dedication**	**Pure challenge**	**Life style integration**	**Entrepreneurship**
6 points	7 points	6 points	5 points	7 points	6 points	4 points	7 points	8 points
14 words	13 words	17 words	4 words	6 words	8 words	16 words	7 words	21 words
Acme	Morality	Self-regulation and self-esteem	Physics and abstract concepts	acknowledgement	Result	Wealth	Family	Power

Needs: 17 + 4 + 6 + 16 = **43 words**, **Values:** 8 + 7 + 21 = **36 words** and **Competencies:** 14 + 13 + 21 = **48 words**.

Table 5. Average values according to the method of "Career anchors" in groups of undergraduates and master's degree students

groups of undergraduates and students / career anchors	**intramural undergraduates of Academy of humanities and pedagogy**	**extramural undergraduates of Academy of humanities and pedagogy**	**intramural students of Academy of humanities and pedagogy**	**extramural students of Academy of humanities and pedagogy**	**Students of VSUES***
Professional competence	5,49	**5,59**	*5,06*	5,4	4,13
Management	*6,09*	6,28	6,14	6,14	**7,59**
Autonomy	6,91	7,13	*6,35*	6,85	**7,19**
The stability of the place of residence	4,87	4,74	4,79	4,78	**6,2**
The stability of the place of work	7,5	**7,84**	7,46	7,65	6,2
Sense of service/dedication	*7,87*	**8,37**	8,34	8,2	6,19
Pure challenge	*5,64*	**5,92**	5,69	5,74	6,07
Life style integration	7,29	**7,83**	*7,13*	7,5	7,28
Entrepreneurship	5,95	6,18	*5,67*	5,96	**7,47**
Average score	6,4	**6,65**	*6,29*	6,47	6,48

VSUES* – Vladivostok state University of Economics and service

For diagnose students ‘self-presentation strategies, we used the method “Scale of measurement of self-presentation tactics” (S. Lee, B. Quigley, etc. 1999). Let’s study the relationship between career orientations and self-presentation strategies (Table 6).

As can be seen from Table 6, the strategy of self-depreciation significantly negatively correlates with such career anchors as management ($r = -0.18$ at $p \leq 0.05$), challenge ($r = -0.21$ at $p \leq 0.01$) and entrepreneurship ($r = -0.17$ at $p \leq 0.05$). Power influence is significantly correlated with management as a career anchor ($r = 0.16$ at $p \leq 0.05$), that is, respondents who have high indicators on the strategy of power influence are often focused on managing other people in their careers. Attractive behavior significantly correlates with the stability of the workplace ($r = 0.16$ at $p \leq 0.05$), that is, the stability of the workplace is important for young people with higher indicators of the strategy of attractive behavior.

Holland’s Personality Types Questionnaire

Consider the relationship between the severity of Shane’s career anchors and Holland personality types. because career anchors are features of motivation, and the type of personality, rather, an individual-psychological feature, the relationship is unlikely. However, in individual features can be shown inclinations as features of motivation. For example, a young man of a social type in the Holland questionnaire often prefers Sense of service or dedication all other career anchors in E. Shane.

As can be seen from Table 7, significant correlations were found only between the realistic type of personality according to Holland and the stability of the place of residence ($r = 0.16$ at $p \leq 0.05$), entrepreneurship ($r = -0.17$ at $p \leq 0.05$). However, interesting results were obtained on the trends of reliable communication. Thus, entrepreneurship is negatively correlated with research and artistic types according to Holland, management-with realistic ($r = -0,12$) and research ($r = -0,11$) types. In addition, the artistic type by Holland correlates with autonomy ($r = 0.11$) as a career anchors.

Table 6. Correlations between career anchors and self-presentation strategies (sample of 163 people)

Self-presentation strategies	Evasion	attractive behavior	Self-exaltation	Self-deprecation	power influence
Professional competence	-0,003	-0,078	-0,094	-0,101	0,056
Management	-0,097	0,061	-0,025	*-0,179*	*0,159*
Autonomy	0,101	-0,083	-0,038	-0,018	0,080
The stability of the place of residence	0,126	0,017	0,033	0,133	0,002
The stability of the place of work	0,138	*0,162*	0,057	0,096	0,09
Sense of service/ dedication	0,039	0,064	-0,047	-0,045	-0,062
Pure challenge	-0,085	0,065	-0,079	**-0,21***	0,108
Life style integration	0,046	0,026	-0,001	-0,031	0,060
Entrepreneurship	-0,032	0,019	0,008	*-0,168*	0,111
Average score	-0,003	-0,078	-0,094	-0,101	0,056

* in **bold** and *italics* marked statistically significant correlations on Pearson [https://statpsy.ru/pearson/tablica-persona/] when $p \leq 0.01$, in italics –when $p \leq 0.05$

Table 7. Correlations between career anchors and personality types according to Holland (sample of 163 people)

Prof. personality types	Realistic	Research	Artistic	Social	Enterprising
Professional competence	0,08	0,10	0,08	0,07	0,03
Management	*-0,12**	*-0,11**	-0,07	-0,01	0,09
Autonomy	0,10	0,09	*0,11**	0,10	0,03
The stability of the place of residence	*0,16*	0,06	0,08	0,09	0,01
The stability of the place of work	0	0,03	-0,01	0,06	0,05
Sense of service/ dedication	0,01	0,05	0,04	0,04	0,02
Pure challenge	*-0,13**	-0,10	-0,09	-0,05	0,04
Life style integration	-0,01	-0,02	-0,02	0	-0,01
Entrepreneurship	**-0,17**	*-0,12**	*-0,13**	-0,10	-0,05
Average score	0,08	0,10	0,08	0,07	0,03

* in **bold** and *italics* indicates statistically significant Pearson correlations [https://statpsy.ru/pearson/tablica-persona/] when $p \leq 0.01$, in italics-when $p \leq 0.05$, *italicized with* * – reliable communication trends.

Based on the results obtained, it is possible to design an individual corrective strategy to clarify the career anchors of students. For example, in the above cases, the main direction of corrective action for a second-year student and a first-year master's student will be to work on the awareness of their own desire for autonomy, while for a third – year student-to clarify the desire for competition, competition and the realization of their own career goals in conditions of uncertainty. Thus, the method of chain free associations in combination with the questionnaire "Career anchor" by E. Shane opens up opportunities for learning the unique inner world of each individual, including in the field of career attitudes and expectations.

As a result of an empirical study, a lower degree of orientation to the stability of the place of residence was revealed with a high orientation to the stability of the place of work of Crimean students. This may indicate that students and undergraduates of the Pedagogy and Humanities Academy are less likely to seek competence in their careers (Professional competence, Management and Entrepreneurship), while there is an emotional oversupply about the career anchors of needs (Autonomy, Security - the stability of the place of residence and Pure challenge), thus we can talk about an intrapersonal conflict. It can be concluded that the desire to change the place of residence is based on a contradictory desire for autonomy, security and pure challenge. That is, the desire to leave your hometown to build a career in the chosen direction may be related to the manifestation of career anchors' needs, or lack of career anchors of competence.

REFERENCES

Ahmed, Azza. (2014). Self-Presentation Strategies among Users of Social Networking Sites. *International Journal of Interactive Communication Systems and Technologies*, *4*, 64-78. 10.4018/IJICST.2014070105.

Alavi, S. B., Moteabbed, S. & Arasti, M. R. (2012). "A qualitative investigation of career orientations of a sample of Iranian software engineers". *Scientia Iranica.*, *19*(3), 662–673. doi:10.1016/j.scient. 2011.08.033.

Golenkova, L. A. & Chernyaeva, V. V. (2013). "Specifics of career settings in students of higher educational institutions." *Fundamental research*. No. 6–4. pp. 1017–1021; URL: http://fundamental-research. ru/ru/article/view?id=31683 (accessed 25.01.2019).

Igbaria, Magid. & Greenhaus, Jeffrey. & Parasuraman, Saroj. (1991). "Career Orientations of MIS Employees: An Empirical Analysis". *MIS Quarterly.*, *15*, pp. 151–169. 10.2307/249376.

Ivanova, N. A. (2013). "Application of the method of free associations in empirical sociological research." *Vestnik SPbSU. Ser.* 12. Vol. *3*, pp. 116–122.

Kaplan, D. M. (2014). "Career anchors and paths: The case of Gay, Lesbian, Bisexual workers" *Human Resource Management Review*, Vol. *24*, № 2. pp. 119–130.

Lazarova, M., Cerdin, J. L. & Liao, Y. (2014_. "The Internationalism Career Anchor" *International Studies of Management & Organization*, Vol. *44*, № 2. pp. 9–33.

Lee, S., Quigley, B. M., Nesler, M. S., Corbett, A. B. & Tedeschi, J. T. (1999). Development of a self-presentation tactics scale. *Personality and Individual Differences*, *26*, 701-722.

Lozhechkina, A. D., Bakunova, I. V. & Tkachenko, A. V. (2017). "Dynamics of career scenarios of University students with different professionalization". *International research journal*, № *04* (58). Part 2. pp. 156-161. DOI: https://doi.org/10.23670/IRJ.2017.58.134.

Markin, V. N. (2011). "Determinanty formirovaniya individual'noi kar'ernoi strategii [Determinants of Individual Career Strategy Formation]". *Social psychology and society*, № *4*. pp. 27–49.

Meshcheryakov, B. G. & Zinchenko, V. P. (2007). *Large psychological dictionary*. SPb. Prime-EUROZNAK, 672, [6] p. (Large University library).

Mogilevkin, E. A. & Novgorodov, A. S. (2011). "Research of leading motives of career self-determination in University students". *Territory of new opportunities. Bulletin of Vladivostok state University of Economics and service*. No. *1* (10). pp. 61–78.

Rodrigues, R., Guest, D. & Budjanovcanin, A. (2013). "From anchors to orientations: Towards a contemporary theory of career preferences". *Journal of Vocational Behavior*, Vol. *83*, pp. 142–152.

Schein, E. H. (1996). "Career anchors revisited: implications for career development in the 21st Century" *The Academy of Management Executive*, Vol. *10*, № 4. pp. 80–88.

Schein, E. H. & Van Maanene, J. (2016). "Career anchors and job/role planning: Tools for career and talent management. *Organizational Dynamics*, Vol. *45*, Iss. 3. pp. 165–173.

Starikov, P. A. (2013). "Method of complex analysis of semantic associations in the study of the "creative ethos" of modern student youth". *Education and science*, No. *7* (106). pp. 114–125.

Ternovskaya, O. P. (2006). *Features of career orientations of students at the final stage of higher education*. autoref. dis. on competition of a scientific degree of the candidate of psychology science (19.00.07 – age and pedagogical psychology). M. 20 pp.

Volkova, N. V. & Chiker, V. A. (2016). "Osobennosti kar'ernoj motivacii v kontekste teorii pokolenij: rezul'taty jempiricheskogo issledovanija [Features of Career Choices through the Generation Theory: The Results of Empirical Research]". Vestnik of Saint Petersburg University. Ser. 8. *Management*, 2016, issue 4, pp. 79-105.

Volkova, N. V. & Chiker, V. A. (2018). "Career aspirations of undergraduates studying at some strategic occupational programs". *Sotsial'naia psikhologiia i obshchestvo* [*Social Psychology and Society*], Vol. 9, no. 1, pp. 90-107. doi:10.17759/sps.2018090107 (In Russ., abstr. in Engl.).

Volkova, N. V. & Chiker, V. A. (2016). "Features of Career Choices through the Generation Theory: The Results of Empirical Research. Vestnik of Saint Petersburg University. Ser. 8. *Management*, issue *4*, pp. 79-105.

Volkova, V. P. & Glushach, N. N. (2016). "Differences in understanding career development in the intergenerational aspect". *Paper presented at* the *International scientific and practical conference of the humanitarian foundations of social progress: Russia and modernity: collection of articles*, Moscow, Russia, April 25-27.

Volkova, N. V. & Chiker, V. A. (2018). "Career aspirations of undergraduates studying at some strategic occupational programs" *Social psychology and society*. 9.1, 90-107. doi:10.17759/ sps. 2018090107.

In: Psychological Service … ISBN: 978-1-53618-160-9
Editor: Svitlana V. Kucherenko

Chapter 5

RESEARCH OF THE UNIVERSITY PSYCHOLOGICAL SERVICE: PECULIARITIES OF ATTENTION PARAMETERS AND THEIR DYNAMICS IN 17-23-YEAR-OLD FEMALE STUDENTS

Eugene Y. Brunner*[*]*, PhD
Psychology Department,
V.I. Vernadsky Crimean Federal University,
Yalta, Crimea, Russia

ABSTRACT

The article deals with the dynamics of attention parameters of 916 17-23-year-old girls during a 5-min work with a proofreading test based on Landolt's ophthalmologic rings. The mean normative data of certain parameters are obtained as well as their regular patterns and peculiarities of correlation relationships. The factors that lead to decline and

---

[*]Corresponding Author's Email: brunner_eu@mail.ru.

improvement of attention are discussed, looking into the mechanisms of interrelation between working speed and attention parameters.

Keywords: voluntary attention, dynamics of attention parameters, proofreading test

INTRODUCTION

The problem of study of human cognitive sphere is one of the most relevant and important problems in modern psychology, for the data of cognitive processes significantly widen our perception of human potential. Without any doubt we can state that attention in particular plays a great role in human mental activity. As certain authors specify, it is a universal non-specific basis for any successfully running psychological process (Rusalov and Mekachchi 1973). In addition, attention, along with memory and imagination, is referred to as the so-called universal cross-cutting mental processes. Together, these processes form the axis of "psychic time", where the "psychic present" corresponds to attention, while memory and imagination define the "psychic past" and "psychic future", respectively (Vekker 1998).

Attention is one of the most important psychological functions, which provides for the optimization of practically any human activity, for a person's interaction with the world around, for the processes of upbringing, education and professional activity. Attention parameters, alongside with other processes, personal characteristics and peculiarities of psychological states, are of principal significance for vocational selection as well as for diagnostics of functional deviations in brain activity.

The identification of leading parameters of attention is equally important for attention research (Brunner 2018). The overwhelming majority of the researchers from soviet school of psychological thought recognizes as the main experimentally identifiable attention parameters such basic ones as *stability* (constancy, sustainedness), *shiftability* (switching), *concentration* (undistracted, undivided attention), *span* and *distribution* (Breslava 1999, 145; Dobrynin 1972; Rubinshtein 1998, 425-421; Strakhov 1969; et al.). According to I. V. Dubrovina et al. these parameters can be present in any type of attention (Dubrovina, Danilova and Prikhozhan 1999, 143-156).

Along with the basic ones, some authors also distinguish such attention parameters as *selectivity* (Chun, Golomb and Turk-Browne 2011, 75-76; Cohen 2014, 306-307; Coull 1998; Duncan 1984; James 1890; Kahneman 1973, 201; Luria 2006; Oades 1995, 428; Wickens and McCarley 2008, 2; et al.), *focusing* (Bukhanovsky, Kutyavin and Litvak 2003, 137), intensity (strain, grade, depth) (Bukhanovsky, Kutyavin and Litvak 2003, 137; Falikman 2006, 97; Gippenreiter 1983; Jakow 2006, 1146; Uznadze 2004, 346; et al.), *objectness* (object-based attention) (Anderson 2002, 99-102; Baylis and Driver 1993; Behrmann, Zemel, and Mozer 1998; Duncan 1984; Egly, Driver, and Rafal 1994; Posner et al. 1985; Rock and Guttman 1981; et al.), *absorption* (Dormashev and Romanov 1995, 16-17; Falikman 2006, 36; Spielberger 2004, 244, 257, 557, 707; et al.), *accommodation* and *inertia* (Titchener 1910, 293-299), *constancy, lability, adaptation speed* (Uznadze 2004, 346), elasticity (Gippenreiter and Romanov 2005, 98), *immersion* (preoccupation in activity, self-absorption) (Bukhanovsky, Kutyavin, and Litvak 2003, 137, 139), *mobility* (Strakhov 1969, 14; Tarasova 1999, 50; et al.) or *maneuverability* (Tarasova 1999, 50).

It is evident that as well as any other regulated psychic process the voluntary attention is characterized by a fluctuating dynamics, in which periods of high concentration interlace with periods of relatively low concentration. These fluctuations, as some scientists state (Vaganyan et al. 2008), happen under the influence of external circumstances; they also depend on the state of the organism itself and on physiologo-biochemical oscillative processes running on different organizational levels of a living system.

Attention processes are very sensitive to different functional states, e.g., to fatigue and strain (Charykova 2009). We can model such fatigue and strain on the basis of monotonous activity, e.g., a proofreading test. From our point of view, it will be interesting not only to get mean normative data of these or those attention parameters, but also to study the peculiarities of their dynamics. Such a study will highlight special features of this or that parameter and certain regular patterns of the fluctuation process in general.

Taking into consideration all the above-mentioned, we specify our research target as peculiarities of attention parameters and the research subject as the dynamics of voluntary attention parameters in 17-23-year-old girls in the process of monotonous work.

METHODS

Participants

To investigate the attention parameters in this research we used a formsheet for the proofreading test based on Landolt's ophthalmologic rings, in which a testee had to cross out three symbols in three different manners. The experiment as such lasted for 5 min. Every 30 sec the experimenter pronounced the word "Line". On the basis of the processing the raw data, such as the number of worked out, correctly and erroneously crossed out signs, as well as missed ones, we calculated such parameters as working speed (productivity), accuracy, thinking productivity, attention concentration, volume of visual information, information processing speed, intellectual work capacity and efficiency of work. Thus, in the course of the research, processing the raw data, we got attention parameters by ten 30-sec intervals.

The described technique is interesting in the aspect that it can be applied as early as from the age of six (Nemov 1998, 173-179). In addition, the subjects do not get used to stimulus material, since it is rather difficult to remember the location of ring breaks. If necessary, the problem of remembering or the novelty of the stimulus can be solved in a very simple way — the experimenter just has to rotate the form in order to present to the testee another (one of the four) side of the sheet.

The undoubted advantage of the stimulus material based on E. Landolt's rings is that the results obtained with the described technique are easily comparable. We are talking not only about different age groups, but also about subjects who speak different languages, or even illiterate, etc. Another advantage of the technique is that exercising has practically no effect on the results of the proofreading test, and therefore it can be carried out repeatedly. Thus, formsheets with rings can be used in research even when, according to the conditions of the experiment, frequent use of the technique is necessary.

The formsheet of the technique shows a sequence of rings arranged row by row in random order. In total, you can find eight types of rings in the form: four rings with left-right and up-down breaks, and four types of rings with diagonal breaks (Brunner 2006; Brunner 2012). The height of the ring is usually equal to the height of the capital letter printed with the 14 font size.

In order to make the testees better understand and follow the given instructions, the first row of the modified by us formsheet is separated from the rest with a horizontal line. In our instructions, we call it a template row. This row is convenient to make notes on, e.g., you can mark there which rings and in what way you have to cross out.

For the convenience of processing and interpretation in our research we adhere to the following data processing algorithm.

At the initial stage, we process the formsheet completed by the testee and enter the raw data t, N, Σ, P, O into the table (see Table 1), where t is the time of the task completion in seconds; N is the number of signs in the worked out part of the table; Σ is the number of correctly crossed out signs; P is the number of missed signs; O is the number of erroneously crossed out signs; $P+O$ is the total number of erroneous actions.

It is important to point out that if the terms of experiment expect the testee to cross out different types of signs in different ways, then during processing two kinds of erroneous actions can be taken into account separately: when the wrong sign is crossed out or when the desired sign is crossed out, but not in the way indicated in the instruction.

At the second stage, we calculate such parameters as n — the number of signs that had to be crossed out, and M — the total number of crossed out signs, according to the following formulae:

Table 1. Processing the results of proofreading experiment

№	Note	t, sec	Raw data (number of signs)							Attention parameters					
			N	Σ	P	O	P + O	n	M	A, *signs per sec*	T, *conventional units*	E, *signs*	K, %	V, *bits*	etc.
1															
…															
n															
Total per experiment															
Mean per batch															

$$n = \Sigma + P \text{ and } M = \Sigma + O.$$

We also enter these parameters into the corresponding columns of the summary table.

At the third stage, after entering the primary data into the table, the actual processing and calculation of attention parameters begins:

- *Productivity* of attention (**A**, *signs per sec*) during the task completion:

$$A = \frac{N}{t};$$

- *Accuracy* of work (**T**, *conventional units*, the calculation accuracy is 0.01):

$$T_2 = \frac{\Sigma}{n};$$

- *Coefficient of thinking productivity* or *the degree of accuracy of the task fulfillment* (**E**, *signs*, the accuracy of the calculations is

1.0), which shows how many viewed symbols were correctly perceived and is often used in perception studies:

$$E_2 = N \cdot T_2;$$

- *Intellectual work capacity* $\boldsymbol{A_{yp}}$ (*signs per sec*):

$$A_{yp} = \frac{N}{t} \cdot \frac{M-(O+P)}{n};$$

- level of *attention concentration* (***K***, *%*):

$$K = \frac{\Sigma - P - O}{n} 100\% \; ;$$

- *quality of work* or *its efficiency* (***R***, *%*):

$$R = \left(1 - \frac{P+O}{N}\right) \cdot 100\%;$$

- *volume of visual information* (***V***, *bits*):

$$V = 0.5936 \cdot N,$$

where

0.5936 is the average amount of information per character (*bits*);

- *visual information processing speed* (or an indicator of productivity and stability of attention) (***Q***, *bits per sec*):

$$Q = \frac{V - 2.807 \cdot (P+O)}{t},$$

where

V is the amount of visual information (*bits*) per time *t* (*sec*); *2.807* bits is the loss of information per missed sign.

At the final stage of data processing, grounding on the results obtained for parameters *P, O, P+O, n, M, A, T, E, K, R,* A_{yp}, *V* and *Q*, we built graphs that clearly reflect the dynamic changes in these attention parameters for each 30-second period of time.

The potential for use of the proof reading test based on E. Landolt's ophthalmologic rings is much wider than we have shown in this paper. As for methodology and organization of research with various techniques for assessing the attention parameters of people of different ages, as well as for assessing the influence of various factors on these parameters, we have already described them earlier (Brunner 2006; Brunner 2012; Brunner and Mizin 2013).

The research was carried out at Crimean State Institute of Humanities. The students' group examination was carried out amid familiar surroundings, in classrooms. The test data were processed with the help of the statistic packet *Statistica for Windows (ver. 8.0).* The difference between the studied parameters was estimated with Student's t–test by $P < 0.05$. The correlation analysis was carried out using Spearman's rank correlation coefficient.

Results and Discussion

To analyze the attention peculiarities we studied a sample group of 916 girls at the age of 17-23. The received in the research mean values of attention parameters for 300-sec work with the proofreading test are displayed in Table 2.

The dynamics of the obtained in the research mean values of attention parameters for each 30-sec interval are displayed in Figure 1-8. The dotted line on coordinate graphs signifies the mean value of the parameter under consideration, along the vertical axis we marked the values of a certain parameter and along the horizontal one — the series number.

The presented illustrations reveal the identity of dynamics patterns of such parameters as A, E_2, V, Q, A_{yp}. The graphs evidently show that after the first 30 sec of work the mean values of these parameters significantly fell down, then we observe their rapid growth (Series 2-4) and equalization with small fluctuations near the mean value (Series 5-9). After 210 sec of relative stabilization, as one can see from the graphs, the mean values of attention parameters grow (Series 10).

Table 2. Mean values of attention parameters of 916 17-23-year-old girls

Parameters		Mean Values ± Std. Dev.
A	Productivity (*signs per sec*)	11,5 ± 4,6
T_2	Accuracy (*conventional units*)	9,1 ± 0,8
E_2	Thinking productivity (*signs*)	314,7 ± 133,7
K	Attention concentration (%)	793,3 ± 222,6
V	Volume of visual information (*bits*)	204,2 ± 82,1
Q	Information processing speed (*bits per sec*)	5,5 ± 2,9
A_{yp}	Intellectual work capacity (*signs per sec*)	9,5 ± 4,6
R	Efficiency of work (%)	956,7 ± 48,6

Applying Student's t–test revealed that the initial lowering (Series 2), the successive growth (Series 3-4) and fluctuations of all the above-mentioned parameters displayed statistically significant difference compared to the initial level. This fact points out that a person needs about a minute to get into the working process. The following dynamics shows that the mean values of parameters equalize from the fourth to the ninth series and after that they start to grow.

It is worth noting that there is a statistically significant difference between the mean values of all the described parameters in the first and second series from one side and their mean values in all the following series from the other.

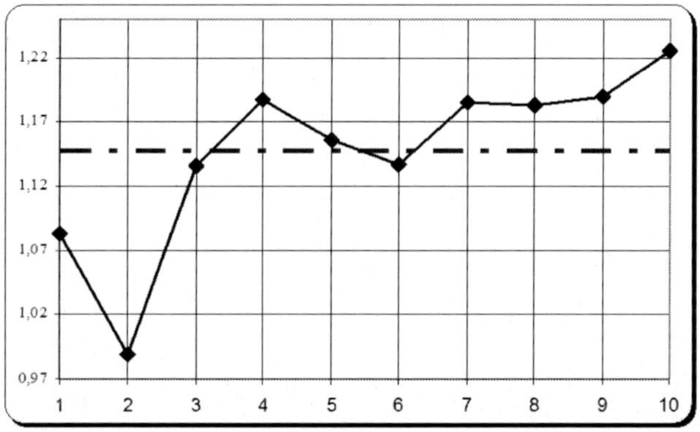

Figure 1. The dynamics of the working speed or productivity (***A**, signs per sec*).

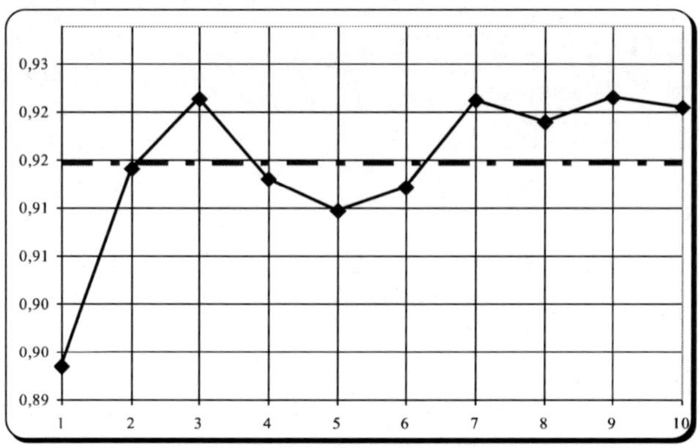

Figure 2. The dynamics of the accuracy ($\boldsymbol{T_2}$, *conventional units*).

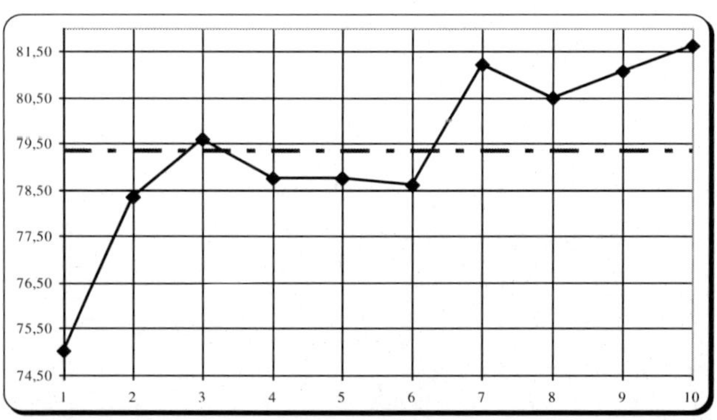

Figure 3. The dynamics of the level of attention concentration (***K***, %).

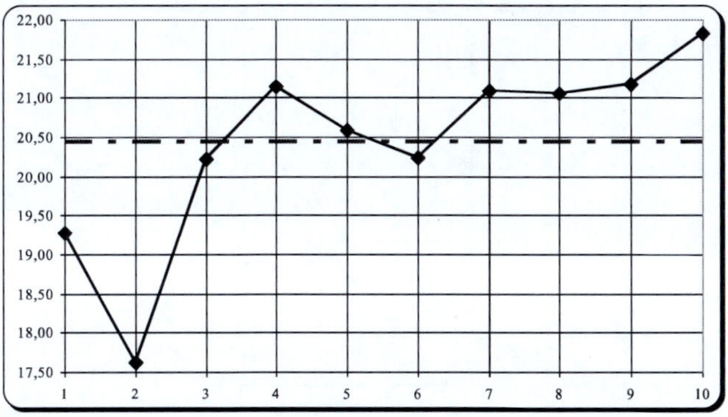

Figure 4. The dynamics of the volume of visual information (***V***, *bits*).

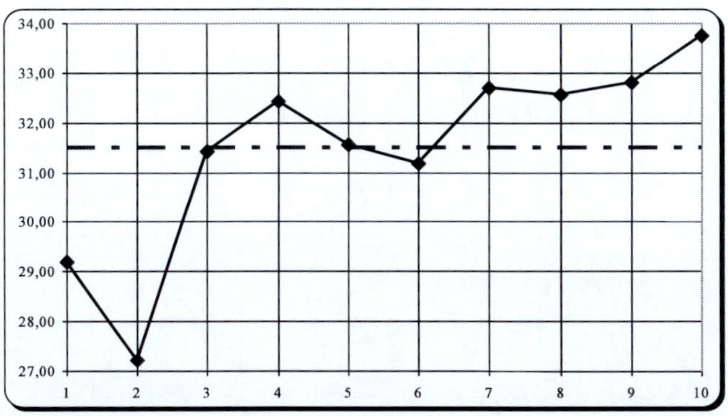

Figure 5. The dynamics of the thinking productivity or grade of accuracy in task fulfillment ($\boldsymbol{E_2}$, *signs*).

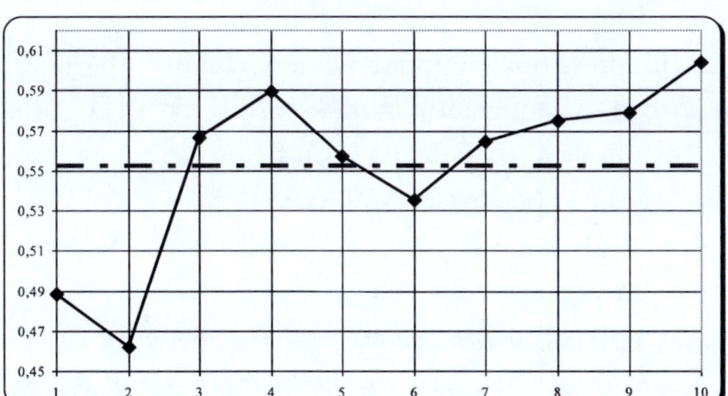

Figure 6. The dynamics of the visual information processing speed or productivity and stability of attention (***Q***, *bits per sec*).

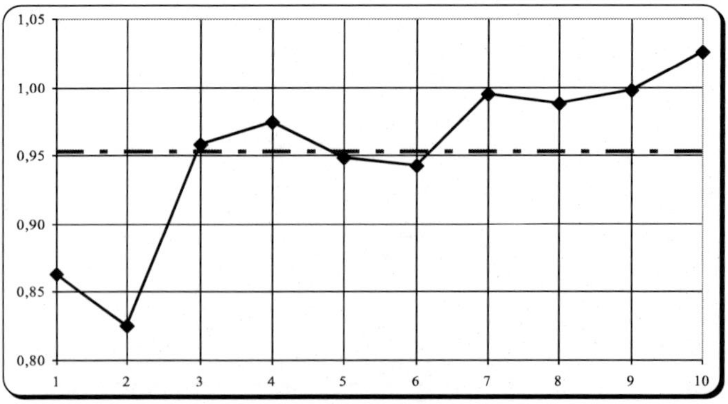

Figure 7. The dynamics of the intellectual work capacity (***A**$_{yp}$*, *signs per sec*).

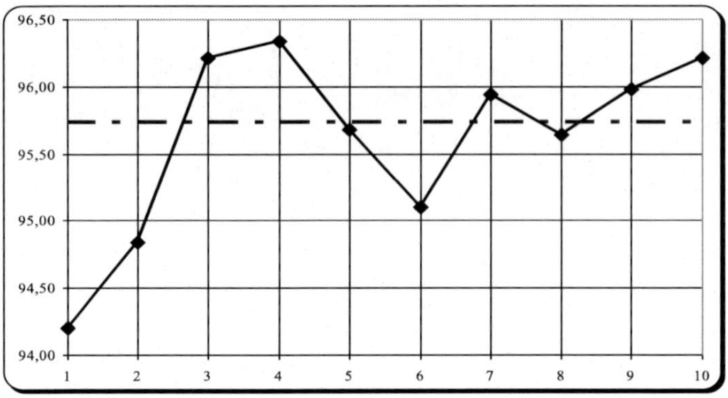

Figure 8. The dynamics of the quality (efficiency) of work (***R**,* %).

A slightly different dynamics of the mean values is observed in parameters T_2 (Figure 2), K (Figure 3) and R (Figure 8). As distinct from the above-described dynamics of parameters A, E_2, V, Q, A_{yp} after 30 sec of work the testees showed statistically significant growth in accuracy (by 2,3%, [$t = -4{,}35$; $P < 0{,}0001$]), concentration (by 4,45%, [$t = -2{,}95$; $P < 0{,}003$]) and statistically non-significant growth in efficiency of work (by 0,67%). In the succeeding series, up to the ninth one, we observed the similarity in patterns of these graphs and the patterns of all the other parameters. However, in Series 10, on the background of the growth of all the other parameters, the accuracy of work displayed a statistically non-significant lowering by 0,12%, while concentration and efficiency of work showed a statistically non-significant growth by 0,69% and 0,24% correspondingly.

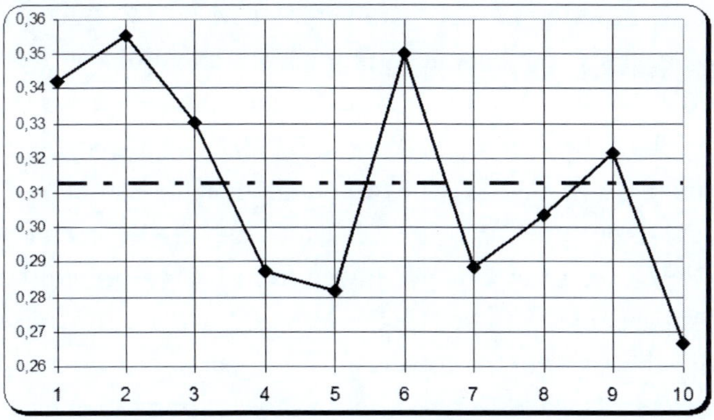

Figure 9. The dynamics of the number of erroneously crossed out signs (***O***, *signs*).

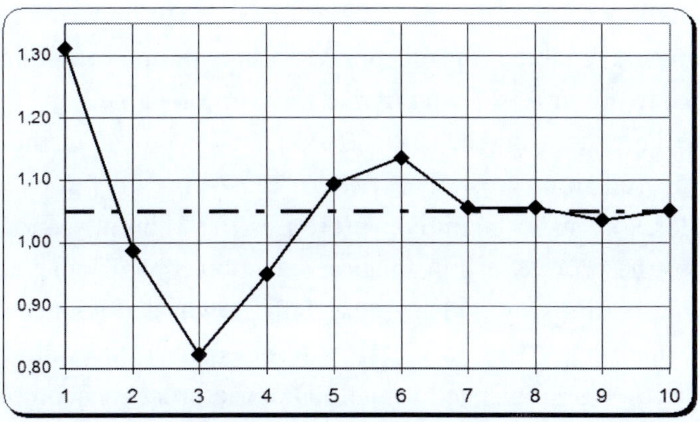

Figure 10. The dynamics of the number of missed signs (***P***, *signs*).

Taking into consideration that such parameters as the number of erroneously crossed out and missed signs were used in calculation of certain attention parameters, we have to get at the specific reason for changing, on the one hand, of the accuracy and concentration of attention and of the dynamics of the mean values of the other parameters, on the other. On the following figures the patterns of the dynamics of the number of erroneously crossed out (Figure 9) and missed (Figure 10) signs are displayed.

One can see from the charts that, alongside with the decrease of the working speed in Series 2, such parameters as A, E_2, V, Q, A_{yp} get lower, while the accuracy and concentration of attention grow. This is accompanied by a statistically significant decrease in the number of the missed signs (by 24,6% [t = -5,42; P < 0,0001]) and a statistically non-significant increase (by 3,83%) in the number of the erroneously crossed out signs. At the same time in Series 6, when the mean values of parameters A, E_2, V, Q, A_{yp}, R get lower, we observe growth both in the number of erroneously crossed out and missed signs. In Series 10 the situation with the growth and lowering of the parameters is similar to the situation in Series 2. The difference lies in the fact that in Series 10 one can observe a certain decrease in the mean values of the parameter T_2.

The described processes give grounds for a deduction that in the beginning the lowering of the mean values of the working speed and most other parameters enabled the accuracy, concentration of attention and efficiency of work to rise, which rise was accompanied by the higher focusing of the testees on the task fulfillment. However, in this case the number of missed signs grew. This pattern can be possibly connected with the activation of such cognitive processes as thinking and memory included into the process of information selection. Later comes the period when the role of thinking and memory falls down, actions become more automatic, which leads first to the growth and then to the stabilization of the proofreading working speed as well as of the processes combined with such parameters as E_2, V, Q, A_{yp}. At the period of stability we observe a slightly different pattern of erroneous actions (Figure 9-10): their number synchronically either grows (Series 6) or drops (Series 7).

If the number of errors were connected with just one psychological process providing advertence, at a later stage we would have observed synchronous fluctuations of the number of missed or erroneously crossed out symbols. However, that doesn't happen; in the sequel there comes another phase of desynchronizing in Series 10 compared with Series 9: the number of erroneously crossed out symbols displays a statistically significant drop by 17,0% ([t = -2,45; P < 0,014]) and the number of missed symbols, on the contrary, shows a statistically non-significant rise by 1,6%. At the same time, a statistically significant growth was observed not only in the working speed (by 3,03%, [t = -3,06; P < 0,002]), but also in the mean values of such parameters as E_2 (by 2,92%, [t = -2,80; P < 0,005]), V (by 3,03%, [t = -3,06; P < 0,002]), Q (by 4,31%, [t = -3,03; P < 0,002]), A_{yp} (by 2,80%, [t = -2,05; P < 0,04]), and the parameters K and R, though growing, show only a statistically non-significant rise. Thus, it becomes evident that the quality of erroneous actions is influenced by different mechanisms.

To understand in details similarities and differences in the dynamics patterns we conducted a correlation analysis between the mean values of attention parameters, the results of which are shown in Table 3.

As one can see from the table, between the parameters A, T_2, E_2, K, V, Q and A_{yp}, there is a positive correlation, which points to the fact that the growth of one parameter leads to the growth of the rest of them, and vise versa. As for the accuracy of attention, we can mention that in spite of the absence of its statistically significant correlations with the parameters A, E_2, V, and Q, we still see a stable tendency to the above-mentioned process.

In our opinion, the correlations between the parameter R and other attention parameters are of interest. The revealed pattern shows that the lower working speed is, the higher is its efficiency, which manifests itself in the fact that under such conditions the testees make less errors and their values of the parameters T_2, E_2, K, V, Q and A_{yp} grow.

The values of the correlations of parameters P and O are worth a separate mentioning. The negative values of these parameters speak for their inverse relations with other attention parameters. In other words, the growing number of missed signs has statistically significant connection with the lowering of the accuracy of attention. At the same time, the growing number of erroneously crossed out rings leads to worsening of the values of such parameters as A, E_2, V, Q, A_{yp} and R. The remarkable thing is that the parameters P and O do not have statistically significant correlations with the concentration of attention (K). However, here as well we see a stable tendency to the pattern of the growth of the erroneous actions of the testees combined with the lowering of concentration. All that again points out that namely the number of erroneous actions itself is directly connected with the speed and efficiency of work as well as with the information processing speed, which finally leads to the changing of the level of the testees' advertence. And the main factor influencing the processes, which accompany attention, is not the number of the missed signs, but the number of the erroneously crossed out ones. This fact once again manifests a tight connection between the attention and the processes of thinking and perception.

If we look closely at the erroneous actions in general, we see, as it is clear from the displayed charts (Figure 9-10), that the number of the missed signs at all the stages of work markedly prevails over the number of the erroneously crossed out ones.

As the analysis applying Student's T-test showed, there is a statistically significant difference by 100,1% [t = -2,78; P < 0,0056] between the mean values of the parameters *P* and *O*. However, in spite of that, the number of the erroneously crossed out signs is connected to a greater extent than the number of the missed ones with the process of advertence/inadvertence.

Table 3. Matrix of intercorrelations between the mean values of attention parameters

	Attention parameters								
	O	*A*	T_2	E_2	*K*	*V*	*Q*	A_{yp}	*R*
P	0,14	-0,11	**-0,74***	-0,19	-0,52	-0,11	-0,37	-0,28	-0,22
O		**-0,78***	-0,34	**-0,77***	-0,56	**-0,78***	**-0,78***	**-0,74***	**-0,72***
A			0,46	**0,99***	**0,65***	**1,00***	**0,96***	**0,97***	**-0,70***
T_2				0,56	**0,94***	0,46	0,61	**0,65***	**0,75***
E_2					**0,73***	**0,99***	**0,97***	**0,99***	**0,79***
K						**0,65***	**0,73***	**0,80***	**0,79***
V							**0,96***	**0,97***	**0,79***
Q								**0,97***	**0,75***
A_{yp}									**0,89***

Note. With the sign "*" we marked the significant correlations. For definition of letter symbols please see Table 2.

CONCLUSION

Thus, the received data show that at different periods of the proofreading based on the informationally non-significant symbols the female testees applied different psychological mechanisms and strategies of the information processing. The beginning of the proofreading was connected with the higher concentration and with the testees' orientation towards the accuracy of the task fulfillment, which led to the increase in the efficiency of work and to the lowering of its speed and such parameters as E_2, V, Q, A_{yp}. In addition to the above, the number of the erroneously crossed out signs grew and the number of the missed ones dropped.

Later, when some actions of the testees became automatic, they kept in mind the signs that they had to cross out, there occurred a period of certain stability lasting for 210 sec. Then proceeded an increase in the mean values of the parameters A, K, E_2, V, Q, A_{yp}, R and P, on the one hand, and a decrease in the accuracy and the number of erroneously crossed out signs, on the other one. If the testees continued to work with the proofreading test, we would not rule out the possibility of repeating fall and growth of the parameters. However, as we established, at different periods the testees would make errors of different types. It is connected with the fact that different mechanisms influence the quality of erroneous actions. This issue is subject to further verification. We can only assume that by this kind of activity during the information processing there can appear changes in type of memory (e.g., from operative to short term and/or long term one), level of applied volitional effort, motivation, strategy of the sign finding and information selection, state, as well as quantity of involved psychophysiological resources and level of strain of the nervous system.

In the following works we plan to conduct analysis of gender differences in the dynamics of interrelations between the attention parameters.

Acknowledgment

I wish to express my deep gratitude to all the participants of the experiment.

References

Anderson, J. R. (2002). *Kognitivnaya psikhologiya* [*Cognitive Psychology*]. Saint-Petersburg: Piter. (In Russian).

Baylis, G. C. & Driver, J. S. (1993). "Visual attention and objects: evidence for hierarchical coding of locations." *Journal of Experimental Psychology: Human Perception and Performance, 19*, 451-470.

Behrmann, M., Zemel, R. S. & Mozer, M. C. (1998). "Object-based attention and occlusion: Evidence from normal participants and a computational model." *Journal of Experimental Psychology: Human Perception and Performance, 24*(4), 1011-1036.

Breslava, G. editor. (1999). *Psiholoģijas vārdnīca* [*Dictionary of Psychology*]. Rīga: Mācību grāmata. (In Latvian).

Brunner, E. Yu. (2006). *Luchshe, chem supervnimanie: metodiki diagnostiki i psikhokorrektsii* [*Better than super attention: methods of diagnosis and psychological correction*]. Rostov-na-Donu: Feniks. (In Russian).

Brunner, E. Yu. (2012). "K voprosu metodologii diagnostiki vnimaniya i avtomatizatsii obrabotki dannykh korrekturnoi proby na osnove oftal'mologicheskikh kolets E. Landol'ta. [On the methodology of the attention diagnostics and automatic processing of the data of a proof-correction test based on E. Landolt's ophthalmological rings.]" *Naukovii chasopis NPU im. M. P. Dragomanova, 36*(60), 188-195. (In Russian).

Brunner, E. Yu. (2018). "Mind Mapping in Education: Its Usage in Psychologists' Training as Exemplified by the Educational Module – "Attention Characteristics" *Astra Salvensis*, *2*, 239-260.

Brunner, E. Yu. & Mizin, V. I. (2013). “Grape Polyphenols Attenuate Psychological Stress.” In *Advanced Bioactive Compounds Countering the Effects of Radiological, Chemical and Biological Agents. NATO Science for Peace and Security Series A: Chemistry and Biology*, edited by G. Pierce, V. Mizin and A. Omelchenko, 229-240. Springer, Dordrecht. doi: https://doi.org/10.1007/978-94-007-6513-9_19.

Bukhanovsky, A. O., Kutyavin, Yu. A. & Litvak, M. E. (2003). *Obshchaya psikhopatologiya* [*General psychopathology*]. Rostov-on-Don: Feniks. (In Russian).

Charykova, I. A. (2009). “Dinamika psikhofiziologicheskikh pokazatelei sportsmenov na raznykh etapakh podgotovki.” [Dynamics of the psychophysiologic parameters in sportsmen at different stages of training] *Voennaya meditsina. Minsk, 3*, 133-136. (In Russian).

Chun, M. M., Golomb, J. D. & Turk-Browne, N. B. (2011). “A Taxonomy of External and Internal Attention.” *Annual Review of Psychology, 62*, 73-101.

Cohen, R. A. (2014). “Attention.” In *Encyclopedia of the Neurological Sciences. Second edition*, editors-in-chief: M. J. Aminoff and R. B. Daroff. Vol. *1*, 303-313. Oxford, UK: Elsevier.

Coull, J. T. (1998). “Neural correlates of attention and arousal insights from electrophysiology, functional neuroimaging and psychopharmacology.” *Progress in neurobiology, 55*, 343-361.

Dobrynin, N. F. (1972). “Ob izuchenii svoistv vnimaniya.” In *Voprosy psihologii vnimaniya* [“Study of attention properties.” In *Issues of the psychology of attention*] *4*, 3-17. Saratov: Saratov teaching Institute. (In Russian).

Dormashev, Y. B. & Romanov, V. Y. (1995). *Psikhologiya vnimaniya* [*Psychology of attention*]. Moscow: Trivola. (In Russian).

Dubrovina, I. V., Danilova, E. E. & Prikhozhan, A. M. (1999). *Psikhologiya* [*Psychology*]. Moscow: Academy. (In Russian).

Duncan, J. (1984). “Selective attention and the organization of visual information.” *Journal of Experimental Psychology: General, 113*(4), 501-517.

Egly, R., Driver, J. & Rafal, R. D. (1994). "Shifting visual attention between objects and locations: Evidence from normal and parietal lesion subjects." *Journal of Experimental Psychology: General, 123*(2), 161-177.

Falikman, M. V. (2006). *Obshaya psichologiya* [*General Psychology*], vol. *4*, Attention. Moscow: Academy. (In Russian).

Gippenreiter, Yu. B. (1983). "Deyatel'nost' i vnimanie." In *A. N. Leontiev i sovremennaya psikhologiyaю* ["Activity and attention." In *Leontiev and contemporary psychology*], edited by A. V. Zaporozhets, 165-177. Moscow: Moscow University Press. (In Russian).

Gippenreiter, Yu. B. & Romanov, V. Y., editors. (2005). *Psikhologiya vnimaniya* [*Psychology of attention*]. Moscow: CheRo. (In Russian).

Jakow, D., editor. (2006). *Lexiko tis koinis neoellinikis* [*Dictionary of Standard Modern Greek*] Thessaloniki: Thessaloniki: Institute of Modern Greek Studies, Idrima Manolis Triandafilides Foundation, Thessaloniki Aristotle University. (In Greek).

James, W. (1890). *The principles of psychology*. In two volumes. New York: Henry Holt and company. Vol. *1*.

Kahneman, D. (1973). *Attention and effort*. N. J.: Prentice Hall.

Luria, A. R. (2006). *Lektsii po obshchei psikhologii* [*Lectures on general psychology*]. Saint-Petersburg: Piter. (In Russian).

Nemov, R. S. (1998). *Psikhologiya: Uchebnik dlya studentov vysshikh pedagogicheskikh uchebnykh zavedenii, book 3: Psikhodiagnostika. Vvedenie v nauchnoe psikhologicheskoe issledovanie s elementami matematicheskoi statistiki* [*Psychology: A Handbook for Teachers' Training Colleges, book 3: Psychodiagnosis: Introduction to Scientific Psychological Research, with Elements of Mathematical Statistics*]. Moscow: Vlados. (In Russian).

Oades, R. D. (1995). "Connections between studies of the neurobiology of attention, psychotic processes and event-related potentials." In *Perspectives of Event-Related Potential Research*, edited by G. Karmos, M. Molnar, V. Csepe, I. Czigler, and J. E. Desmedt, 428-438. Amsterdam: Elsevier.

Posner, M. I., Choate, L., Rafal R. D. & Vaughn, J. (1985). "Inhibition of return: neural basis and function" *Cognitive Neuropsychology, 2*, 211-228.

Rock, I. & Guttman, D. (1981). "The effect of inattention on form perception." *Journal of Experimental Psychology: Human Perception and Performance, 7*, 275-285.

Rubinshtein, S. L. (1998). *Osnovy obshchei psikhologii* [*Fundamentals of General psychology*]. Saint-Petersburg: Piter. (In Russian).

Rusalov, V. M. & Mekachchi, L. (1973). "O svyazi ustoichivosti vnimaniya pri rabote s korrekturnoi tablitsei s chastotoi al'fa-ritma fonovoi EEG. [On connection between the attention stability while proofreading and the frequency of alpha rhythm of background electroencephalogram]" *Voprosy psikhologii, 3*, 32-44. (In Russian).

Spielberger, C. D., editor in chief. (2004). *Encyclopedia of applied psychology*. Florida, USA: Elsevier, vol. *1*.

Strakhov, I. V. (1969). "Psikhologicheskaya teoriya vnimaniya." In *Voprosy psihologii vnimaniya* ["Psychological theory of attention." In *Issues of the psychology of attention*] *1*, 3-15. Saratov: Saratov teaching Institute. (In Russian).

Tarasova, L. E. (1999). "*Formirovanie kollektivnogo vnimaniya mladshikh shkol'nikov: obshchepedagogicheskii aspekt.* [*Development of collective attention in junior schoolchildren: a general educational aspect.*]" PhD diss., Saratov. (In Russian).

Titchener, E. D. (1910). *A Text-Book of Psychology*. New York: The Macmillan Company.

Uznadze, D. N. (2004). *Obshaya psichologiya* [*General Psychology*]. Moscow: Smysl; Saint-Petersburg: Piter. (In Russian).

Vahanyan, L. G., Gevorgyan, E. G., Tadevosyan, I. G., Kostanyan, E. G., Tadevosyan, N. E., Maloyan, V. A. & Hayrapetyan, N. A. (2008). "Dinamika pokazatelei vnimaniya v usloviyakh umstvennoi nagruzki. [Dynamics of attention indices in conditions of mental consignment.]" *Meditsinskaya nauka Armenii, 4*, 107-116. (In Russian).

Vekker, L. M. (1998). *Psikhika i real'nost': edinaya teoriya psikhicheskikh protsessov* [*Mind and reality. Unified theory of psychic processes*]. Moscow: Smysl. (In Russian).

Wickens, C. D. & McCarley, J. S. (2008). *Applied attention theory*. Boca-Raton, FL: Taylor & Francis.

In: Psychological Service … ISBN: 978-1-53618-160-9
Editor: Svitlana V. Kucherenko

Chapter 6

RESEARCH OF THE UNIVERSITY PSYCHOLOGICAL SERVICE: B. HELLINGER'S SYSTEMIC CONSTELLATION AS A METHOD OF RESEARCH FOR AN AESTHETIC OBJECT IN THE PROCESS OF STUDYING ART HISTORY

Viktor E. Vynohradov*[1,*]*, PhD
and Eugene Y. Brunner*[2,†]*, PhD
[1]Fine Arts, Teaching Methodology and Design Department,
V. I. Vernadsky Crimean Federal University,
Yalta, Crimea, Russia
[2]Psychology Department,
V. I. Vernadsky Crimean Federal University,
Yalta, Crimea, Russia

* Corresponding Author's Email: vikvin@inbox.ru.
† Corresponding Author's Email: brunner_eu@mail.ru.

Abstract

The article deals with the use of B. Hellinger's family constellations for the study of an aesthetic object as an alternative innovative method in the process of teaching theory and history of art. The experiment was conducted with groups of Art students who had minimal knowledge of the object of study at the time of the experiment. During the constellation process, we studied the artistic features of E. Manet's painting "Le Déjeuner sur l'herbe (The luncheon on the grass)": composition, light effects, colour scheme and plot interactions. As well as the visual study of an object, the constellation process has shown the key role of composition in determining the integral "movement," the "moves" of perception, and the ways of understanding the picture. The insight into the relationship between the influence of the light setting in the picture, its aesthetic transformation, upon the context and scandalous fame of the work was important for the study. The role reception (representative perception) of each character in the painting space was one of the discoveries and the main element of the constellation, which allowed a deeper understanding of the overall concept of the work, its innovative position in the art history.

Keywords: B. Hellinger's systemic constellation, aesthetic objects, painting, perception, representative perception, "Le Déjeuner sur l'herbe (The luncheon on the grass)", Edouard Manet

Introduction

The art of the XIX – early XX centuries, being contradictory, semantically diverse, rich in sign systems of different cultures, ornamental forms of various traditions, aroused the interest of many researchers who tried to reveal the main criteria for the perception of an artistic image, the communicative means of works of art influence upon the viewer, and many other aspects. R. Arnheim, in contrast to Freud, stated that art is a process of knowledge. According to him, the main danger that threatens art is the loss of understanding of art. "We have neglected the gift of comprehending things through our senses. Concept is divorced from percept, and thought moves among abstractions. Our eyes have been reduced to instruments with which to identify and to measure; hence we suffer the paucity of ideas that can be expressed in images and an incapacity to discover the meaning in what we see" (Arnheim 1954, 1).

Interpretation of images, plots, and the variety of author's ideas in works of art has generated many methods of study, such as iconographic, iconological, semiotic, psychoanalytic, historical and cultural, etc. The specific character of these methods is not a source of exhaustive information about the context of the work. Modern research requires a comprehensive art approach to the study and the introduction of interdisciplinary techniques. Among the art studying disciplines the psychology of art is distinguished by its original methodological base that allows one to obtain results not only with the help of the traditional art analysis, but also with the use of an integrated approach to research, involving scientists from various fields.

The study of works of art in the educational process is especially important for creating a holistic picture of the spiritual and material culture interaction, understanding the important role of the creator in the process of materialization of philosophical and aesthetic views. In this regard, A. N. Leont'ev, speaking about works of art, wrote: "As for aesthetic activity, aesthetic creative activity creates namely ideal products – works of art, aesthetic objects... Thus, every product of aesthetic activity is addressed to a person, to people, it is a product designed to influence people, and already in the very process of its creation, it seems to imply that it will be perceived. Of course, an aesthetic product requires a special kind of perception, namely an aesthetic one" (Leont'ev 1983, 233). The communicative property of art involves perceiving it as a message, which always has its own viewer, reader, listener, who perceives this message as an idea. This message is necessarily personal, transmitted under the influence of personal experience, reflecting the whole range of views of a creative person. "What is the object of reflection? The essence is an object of reflection that requires a very specific form. In short, the function of aesthetic activity, in the hypothesis I am developing, is the discovery of life. Therefore, the content of aesthetic activity is always the process of penetration through the meaning" (Leont'ev 1983, 237). This key phrase by A. N. Leont'ev accurately reflects the nature of comprehension of the work by the person who perceives it. It reveals the essence of our proposed research method, which works with the context of the work, penetrating beyond its meaning. This method is B. Hellinger's systemic constellations. Constellation, in fact, is an experimental, innovative method of working with the content of figurative fine art works and its implementation into educational technologies will serve as an original educational complex for studying the theory of fine art, along with the basic ones.

METHODS

Participants

The authors of the article put forward the hypothesis that systemic constellations can become a method of research, first of all, for the most controversial, infamous, shocking paintings by famous artists. It should be noted that up to the present time, systemic constellations have not been used for working with aesthetic objects, with paintings in particular. An important fact in the hypothesis was that the paintings of famous artists were studied and analyzed mainly by representatives of various art schools, and the circumstances having resulted in scandalous fame of these objects were described. For the study, we chose the painting "Le Déjeuner sur l'herbe (The luncheon on the grass)" by Edouard Manet, which in 1863 received mixed evaluation by the jury of the Paris Salon and by the audience. Not admitted to the exhibition by a strict jury, it was put on display thanks to the Emperor Napoleon III's initiative, who decided to create the Salon des Refusés (exhibition of rejects).

According to the methodology, the facilitator has to possess a broad knowledge of the object under study in historical and analytical aspects. However, to maintain the experimental integrity, a minimum level of knowledge about the work under study is desirable both for the representatives of the characters in the painting and for the audience interacting with the painting. This is necessary in order to avoid pre-tuning the judgments of the characters' representatives and the people interacting with the painting. That is why, the group of student participants did not know in advance what picture was going to be studied.

The next stage was the visual contact of the study participants with the work of art. This contact with the painting was important for forming an emotional impression of the work for each of the group members. An important condition for the results of the constellation was also the fixation of the painting composition scheme by the characters' representatives: the location of the figures in the picture and their plot interaction.

Most of the participants of the constellations were art students, whose age, with rare exceptions, was 17-19 years. At the same time, during the discussion, it also became clear that none of the study participants had previously participated in either psychodrama or constellations. Before starting the work, all participants were shown the painting and told the basic rules of working in the group (Vachkov 2000), the main of which were: mutual respect, lack of criticism, as well as reasonable activity of participants and silence of onlookers.

Then, from among the participants, the representative was selected first for the role of the artist of the painting under study: E. Manet. Then E. Manet's (Artist's) representative chose a place in the space (in the room), from which he would "create" the painting, and took his place. The next step was to choose the characters of the painting and to place them in the space in accordance with the painting's composition. After selecting a representative for a particular character, the Artist stood behind the representative for that character, took him/her by the shoulders, put him/her into the "painting" and verbally designated him/her. The painting itself and the schematic arrangement of representatives in the constellations are shown in Figure 1.

After the composition of the painting was reconstructed in the space, we also selected such figures as the Collector, the Viewer – the artist's (the Paris salon's) contemporary and the Modern Viewer. These figures and the Artist's representative were allowed to spontaneously move in space. The figures-characters of the picture were forbidden to move. During all the constellations, the Collector refused to “enter the painting” and participated at a distance.

After selecting all the representatives, we started the research. For a deeper immersion, each of the participants was asked to describe his/her physiological sensations, starting with the feet, ending with the muscles of the face and head. Then they specified the name of their condition and the leading emotion. After the initial survey of physiological sensations and emotional states, the actual research started. For this, each participant was in turn interviewed about what they were thinking about, how they “got” to that place, what their roles in the composition were, what their motives were, etc. Each time, after a character answered the questions, a survey on the change in feelings was conducted, both in the interviewed character of the picture, and in the rest of the representatives. Then we proceeded with the interviewing the next character in the painting. At the end of the initial work with the characters, we began to work with E. Manet’s representative. After this part of the work, the second survey of the characters-in-the-painting’s representatives was conducted.

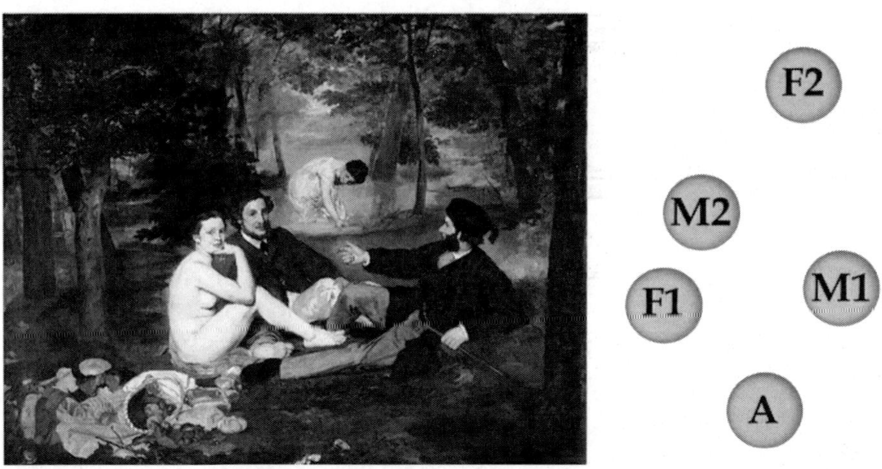

A – Representative of the Artist of the painting, M1 – Male Figure 1, M2 – Male Figure 2, F1 – Female Figure 1, F2 – Female Figure 2.

Figure 1. The picture “Le Déjeuner sur l’herbe (The luncheon on the grass)” and the location scheme of the main representatives.

After completing this part of the work, the Collector, the Viewer of the painting's period and the Modern Viewer were also interviewed.

For didactic and cognitive purposes, art students and other participants sitting around the "painting" were invited to try a role of one of the representatives (physically take the place of a particular figure) or just walk "inside the painting." After that, each of those who both visited the "field" of the painting and took role of one of its characters talked about their feelings, impressions and thoughts that arose when they were at a particular place in the space of the painting.

After the constellation was concluded, the roles were removed from representatives and a final group discussion was held as to what was seen. The carried out work fully corresponded to the methodology of conducting psychodrama (Holmes and Karp 1991; Schutzenberger 2001) and B. Hellinger's systemic constellations (Brunner 2008; Lazorenko 2012; Schlippe and Schweitzer, 2007;Weber 1998).

All stages of working with the painting and group discussion were recorded on a video camera. Then, a shorthand copy of the captured video materials was made as well as their subsequent analysis. In total, three constellations were conducted with different groups of participants and representatives.

RESULTS

In his lecture on the work of E. Manet, M. Foucault (Foucault 2009) compares the attitude to the painting plane (canvas) of Western European artists, starting with the late Renaissance and E. Manet. Unlike its predecessors, who sought to maximize adaptation, fit the canvas into space and context, Manet presents the picture as an object, emphasizes the essential nature of the canvas itself, its aesthetic value. "For Manet, the painting itself is an aesthetic object, which can be viewed from different points of view, under different lighting conditions, and in which one can see the changing art. This is what Michel Foucault considers the beginning of impressionism" (Mardzhi 2019, 57). For our experiment with the content study of the painting "Luncheon on the grass," M. Foucault's line of reasoning about E. Manet's work is interesting for it draws attention to the lighting in the composition. The artist illuminates the group of depicted people with a soft frontal light that matches the natural colour. But at the same time, he also uses an additional source of "plot" light, which helps the viewer to enter the composition and find his/her way around in the context of the plot. The use of several light sources in the composition is found in compositions of different genres by various artists, e. g., in Yuliy Klever's landscapes (Vynohradov 2014, 133), which adds to the works a touch of mystery and the effect of the viewer's presence. The bright lighting of the people depicted in the painting "Luncheon on the grass" from the side of the viewer, and a more contrasting one in the painting "Olympia," caused an unexpected aesthetic effect of "peeping" at the scene. Foucault states that this "…aesthetic transformation can … provoke a moral scandal" (Foucault 2009), revealing an active interaction – the presence of the viewer in the plot of the picture, who seems to illuminate with his/her gaze what is happening in it and is part of it. This interaction practically advantaged the constellation process, since the author himself so to say opened the door to the space of his composition. Deciphering the painting text by the viewer and deciphering it by the group in the process of systemic constellation have only few common aspects. Among the contact points interconnected by interpretation there are the compositional solutions of the painting, the selection of its elements by light and colour, and the internal plot connections of the elements in the composition. The visual assessment of a picture by the viewer was described by N. N. Volkov in his work "Composition in painting." "Understanding the meaning of a painting and the logic of composition can give generalized information about the "integral eye movements," not about actual frequent changes of fixation points, jumps, returns, but about some generalized course of perception of the painting. Imaginary "integral" eye movements reproduce the basis of the composition – its internal connections. These are moves of understanding. ... It is not the eye movements used to reading a verbal text that determine composition, but, on the contrary, composition determines integral "movements," "moves" of perception, moves of understanding" (Volkov 1977, 48). R. Arnheim wrote about the visual perception of a work of art that in structure it represents a sensory analogue of intellectual cognition, and "...the same mechanisms operate on both perceptual and intellectual level, so that terms like concept, judgment, logic, abstraction, conclusion, computation, are needed in describing the work of the senses" (Arnheim 1954, 46).

Table 1. Interrelation of research results in certain areas with aesthetic parameters of the painting

Research areas	Aesthetic parameters of the painting				
	Composition	Lighting	Colour	Plot interactions	Relevance of the concept
1	Collaboration of Nude and clothed figures	Scandalous effect of "peeping" at the scene by the viewer	Contrast of Nude and clothed body	Effects of presence in the picture (male figures) and interaction with the viewer (female figure)	Gender inequality, conflicts of interest, etc.
2	Combining figures from different paintings	Women are united by lighting	Women are united by colour	Kinship of male figures	Detachment
3	Random nature	Naturalness, tension and artificiality	Formality and loneliness	Lack of demand for naturalness	Contrast, heterogeneity
4	Unusual, borrowed, allegorical	Highlighting different topics	Conventional, artificial	Showing different views	Reflecting the era, relevant
5	Close relationship between the disconnected and the lonely	A look at the contemporary	Conditionality of what is happening	The loneliness of nature in the midst of rationalism	Connection of different epochs

In the course of the constellation we investigated such main areas:

1) manifestations of the so-called "scandalousness" of the work;
2) the interactions between the characters in the plot of the painting;
3) reception of each character in the space of the painting;
4) the perception of pictures by the artist, the modern viewer, the collector and the viewer of the Paris Salon époque;
5) the perception of the overall context of the painting, its message in the aesthetic and moral aspects.

Research in these areas has shown, along with random results, clearly formulated sequential concepts worth to present in a Table (Table 1). In the Table, we can trace the interrelation between the studied areas, results and such aesthetic parameters of painting as composition, lighting, colour, plot interactions, relevance of the concept.

DISCUSSION

The main areas of research of an aesthetic object in the course of systemic constellations showed that the progress towards the conceptual basis is associated with a variety of random parameters connected with representatives' reception and personal projections. However, basing on representatives' reception at collective work towards the key topics of those areas, it became possible to recreate a vivid context that logically, realistically and artistically reveals the general concept of the object.

Research in the first area showed that the scandalousness of the paintings manifests itself in the visual perception, formed under the influence of such aesthetic parameters as composition, lighting, colour. The collaboration of Nude and clothed figures evoked a sense of close unity and total disunity at the same time. Highlighting a Nude body with frontal light, with its local academic colour, against the background of officially dressed men, provoked diametrically opposed interpretations. The second female figure standing in the water seemed allegorical to the

Modern Viewer, and pushed the Viewer-Manet's contemporary even closer to a scandalous interpretation.

Research in the second area showed that light and colour in the painting form the plot lines of characters. The female figures were united by lighting and colour, just as the male ones were united by the colour of their clothes. The assumption of the representatives about the kinship of the men really coincided with the fact that the prototypes of the characters in the painting were related to E. Manet. Another assumption that spontaneously appeared during the constellation, that the composition of the "Luncheon on the grass" consists of elements borrowed from different sources, was previously confirmed by art studies. Indeed, it is generally accepted that Raphael's drawing "Judgement of Paris" was the source of the arrangement of the seated figures, and the "Pastoral Concert" by Giorgione or Titian also influenced E. Manet's painting. As a result of representative perception in the constellation, the dominant felt in the painting tendency was the detachment of characters from active interaction.

The third area of research was the representatives' reception, their feelings, reflections and thoughts within and out of the context of the study. Their perception gave results in other areas of research as well. The reflections of the female characters' representatives, who felt their authenticity embodied in nudity and semantic autonomy, were interesting. The naturalness radiated by them did not find proper reactions from phlegmatic men, causing alienation and passive self-sufficiency. Two plot lines caused conflicting feelings.

The fourth research area was the study of the perception of the painting by the Artist, the Modern Viewer, the Collector and the Viewer of the Paris Salon. It is noteworthy that during all the conducted constellations, the Artist's representatives refused "to enter the space of the painting," remaining static during the study. Their reasoning reveals the dominant elements of the composition: despite the fact that female figures are highlighted in colour, the hidden center of the composition is in the male figures. The work reflects the relationship between people in society. Women are secondary and represent a function. The painting became rejected because it depicts the truth, not wanted by society. In general, the composition reveals the theme of idle people's leisure.

The Modern Viewer's reasoning was in line with the Artist's reasoning and, in general, coincided with the Paris Salon Viewer's opinion as well. He/she was paying attention to the woman in the foreground and her gaze. Her impartial gaze suggests that she knows what is happening in the picture. In the Modern Viewer's opinion, the woman was the topic of the men's discussion, she was satisfied with both her functional role and her situation. The Modern Collector believed that the painting was worth buying only because it was created by Edouard Manet. The characters and artistic features of the painting did not appeal to him, and the composition itself caused erotic reflections.

It should be noted that the Nude woman in the foreground of the composition was perceived by the Modern Viewer and the Paris Salon Viewer as an interpreter of the painting content. But it was difficult for them to move further, deeper into the composition, to other images. This fact, as one of the results of the constellation in the fourth area, coincided with E. G. Fisun's interpretation. "A naked Parisian woman on the background of a morning picnic acts as the first object of "looking at," and her very presence causes the subconscious exclusion of all other subjects of the action depicted by E. Manet, since the "erotic gaze" no longer manages to focus on the rest of the painting details" (Fisun 2013, 128). Controlling the gaze of the recipient-viewer is probably one of the main communicative solutions created by E. Manet in his work. A woman (F1), who looks coldly at the viewer, dominates over him, her gaze dictates the behavior of the viewer, and her nakedness shows no hesitation, no desire to appear more beautiful. In his lecture "Point of no return. "Luncheon on the grass" by Edouard Manet" Ilya Doronchenkov claims that this neutral cold piercing look, without the desire to gibbet the onlooker, made the Paris Salon viewer very nervous apart from the nakedness of this woman (Doronchenkov 2018).

The fifth research area was revealed in the discussion of the constellation results, when the perception of the overall context of the picture was formulated by each participant of the study. The scandalous glory of the work was in the bold for its time naked truth about the life of young middle class Parisians. The artist's aesthetic challenge to public opinion and official salon art caused an active rejection of E. Manet's artistic creation.

Conclusion

The experiments conducted by the authors of the article confirm their hypothesis that B. Hellinger's systemic constellations can improve the qualitative parameters of the study of art history material by Art students. They increase the involvement of the audience in the study of the work of art, reveal the peculiarities of the composition, the interaction of the plot elements, the characteristics of the images, visual features and dominant colour solutions. In the course of the constellations, the principles of constructing the "depth" of the picture, its "scene," the planning of the work (the construction of the first, second and subsequent plans of the painting) are discussed and revealed. The plane of a painting turns into a scene having a depth where the representatives of the depicted on it characters stay or move. A "living" painting is a field for the context search. As a result of all this, the constellation helps to formulate the main motive of the work from a new angle.

Thus, B. Hellinger's systemic constellations can become an effective and innovative method for studying works of figurative art in a creative environment. Its use in the educational process requires further research. It is advisable to improve the methodology with a structural approach in selected areas of research, which excludes the possible random judgments of the characters' representatives and random results in general.

Acknowledgment

The authors of the article express their deep gratitude to all the participants of the experiment.

References

Arnheim, R. 1954. *Art and visual perception: A psychology of the creative eye*. Berkeley: University of California Press.

Brunner, E.Yu. 2008. "Tekhnika provedeniya gruppovoi raboty metodom semeinoi sistemnoi terapii po Bertu Hellingeru. [The technique of group work with B. Hellinger's systemic constellations.]" *Problemi suchasnoï pedagogichnoï osviti*. vol. 2. 19:183-195. (In Russian).

Doronchenkov, I. 2018. "*Istorijaiskusstva. "Tochka nevozvrata. "Zavtrak na trave" Jeduarda Mane*" [*Art History. The point of no return. "The luncheon on the Grass" by Edouard Manet*.]" Accessed February 10, 2020 .https://tvkultura.ru/video/show/brand_id/62218/episode_id/2170648/ (In Russian).

Fisun, E.G., 2013. "Modelirovanie prostranstva "zhenskogo" v zhivopisi XIX veka: "muzhskoj vzgljad" i "zhenskoe telo." [Modelling the space of "female" in the XIX century painting: "male gaze" and "female body."]" *Humanitarniy Chasopis* 4:125-130. (In Russian).

Foucault, M. 2009. *Manet and the object of painting*. New York: Tate Pub.

Holmes, P., and Karp, M., editors. 1991. *Psychodrama: Inspiration and Technique*. London: Tavistock/Routledge.

Lazorenko, B.P. 2012. "Kak rabotayut semeinye rasstanovki B. Hellingera v zhiznekonstruirovanii problemnoi molodezhi. [How B. Hellinger's family constellations work in the life-design of troubled youth.]" In *Psikhodrama i sovremennaya psikhoterapiya*. 60–69. Kiev: Institut social'noï ta politychnoï psyhologiï NAPNU; Milenium. (In Russian).

Leont'ev, A.N. 1983. Nekotorye problem psikhologii iskusstva. [Some Problems of Psychology of Art.] In *Izbrannye psikhologicheskie proizvedeniya: v 2 t.* [*Selected psychological works*: in 2 vol.]. Vol. 2. 232-239. Moscow: Pedagogika. (In Russian).

Mardzhi, N.M. 2019. "Eto ne iskusstvo: M. Fuko v poiskakh novykh granei khudozhestvennoi semantiki ["This is not an art": Michel Foucault and new edges of semantics in art]" *Vestnik RGGU. Seriya Filosofiya. Sotsiologiya. Iskusstvovedenie*." 1:54–65. doi: 10.28995/2073-6401-2019-1-54-65 (In Russian).

Schlippe, A. V., and Schweitzer, J. 2007. *Lehrbuch der systemischen Therapie und Beratung* [*Textbook of systemic therapy and counseling*]. Göttingen: Vandenhoeck und Ruprecht.

Schutzenberger, A.P. 2001. *Le Psychodrame* [*Psychodrama*]. Paris: Payot.

Vachkov, I.V. 2000. *Osnovy tekhnologii gruppovogo treninga. Psikhotekhniki* [*Group training technology basics. Psychotechnics*]. Moscow: Os'-89. (In Russian).

Volkov, N.N. 1977. *Kompozitsiya v zhivopisi* [*Composition in painting*]. Moscow: Iskusstvo. (In Russian).

Vynohradov, V. 2014. "Monumental'naya zhivopis' Yu. Klevera v Forosskom dvortse Kuznetsova: khudozhestvennye osobennosti i problema sinteza [Murals of Y. Klever in Kuznetsov'sForos palace: art features and synthesis problem.]" *Vestnik KhGADI*. 1:53-56. (In Russian).

Weber, G., editor. 1998. *Praxis des Familien-Stellens. Beiträge zu systemischen Lösungen nach Bert Hellinger* [*Practice in constellation work. Texts on systemic solutions by Bert Hellinger*]. Heidelberg: Carl-Auer.

In: Psychological Service …
Editor: Svitlana V. Kucherenko ISBN: 978-1-53618-160-9

Chapter 7

RESEARCH OF THE UNIVERSITY PSYCHOLOGICAL SERVICE: VALUABLE AND SEMANTIC ORIENTATIONS OF STUDENTS WITH INTERNET ADDICTION

Irina V. Sultanova*[1,*], *PhD and Olga A. Shutova*[2,†], *PhD
[1]Psychology Department,
Institute of Humanities and Pedagogics of Sevastopol State University,
Sevastopol, Crimea, Russia
[2]Linguodidactics and Foreign Philology Department,
Institute of Humanities and Pedagogics of Sevastopol State University,
Sevastopol, Crimea, Russia

ABSTRACT

The aim of the study was to investigate valuable and semantic orientations of students with Internet addiction. The present empirical study of the features of the system of valuable and semantic orientations

* Corresponding Author's Email: irsan11@rambler.ru.
† Corresponding Author's Email: olgadushina@list.ru.

of high school students with Internet addiction involved 54 undergraduate students. All participants of the study had been selected by means of a cluster sampling method based on the age and education specialty among the students of Sevastopol State University. So the study was conducted on the students male of the 4th year study (20-23 years old) of technical specialty “Computer Science and Computer Engineering” of Sevastopol State University. There is difference in the scale of recognition and respect for people and the influence of others according to the method of S. Bubnova f = 3.481 at the low level, f = 2.046 at the middle level, and f = 1.624 at the high level. Among the addicts, 11 people are on low level, 8 on average one, and 1 on high level, while other students have 3 on low level, 25 on average one, and 6 on high.

In the surveyed sample of 54 students, Internet addiction was detected in 37.04% (20 people) of respondents. The tendency to Internet addiction is observed in 16.67% (9 people) of respondents. The high level of Internet addiction is conected with the peculiarities of the chosen specialtyThe results of the correlation analysis indicate that significant differences in the expression of such values as love, recognition and respect for people and influence on others, and honesty were found among respondents with and without Internet addiction.

Keywords: valuable and semantic orientations, social interaction, Internet addiction, semantic sphere of personality

INTRODUCTION

Valuable orientations of the individual are the main component of his relationship with the society, with himself, and also act as the core of the worldview and the basis of life motivation, activity, and philosophy of life. Valuable and semantic orientations of a person are developed in the process of his social interaction.

The success of socialization primarily depends on how the individual perceives the fundamental values of the environment, social norms, rules, standards, as well as how these components are in harmony with the system of his basic values and meanings.

LITERATURE REVIEW

The problem of the valuable and semantic sphere of personality was studied by such researchers as: K. Abulkhanova-Slavskaya, L. Arkhangelskiy, A. Asmolov, B. Bratus, E. Vasina, L. Vygotsky, A. Zdravomyslov, L. Kogan, L. Lebedev, A. Leont'ev, D. Leont'ev, V. Lisovsky, N. Naumova, M. Rokeach, S. Rubinstein, V. Frankl, A. Khuziakhmetov, M. Yanitsky, and others.

There are many factors that have both as positive as negative influence on the system of valuable and semantic orientations of the individual. One of the negative factors contributing to the decrease in productive social activity, distortion of the process of adequate formation of the valuable and semantic sphere is pathological fascination with computer technologies and Internet resources.

At the present stage of society development the global information environment provides great opportunities for solving a great variety of tasks (communication, leisure, business, etc.). But it is worth to note that information environment, especially the Internet, is a factor that contributes to the development and formation of Internet-dependent behavior. The most exposed to the negative impact of the Internet are students, due to the need to constantly use Internet resources in order to obtain additional information resources. In some cases, this factor can lead to Internet addiction.

Internet addiction contributes to the distortion of the valuable and semantic sphere of students' personality, which can cause social isolation, infantile, excessive lability or fading in the emotional sphere, as well as the formation of difficulties in learning, creating a family, building a career, etc.

Today, the problem of Internet addiction and its impact on a person seems to be quite popular, but still poorly studied.

Theoretical and practical aspects of Internet addiction were studied by such scientists as: A. Voiskunsky, A. Goldberg, T. D. Goldsmith (Goldsmith 2000), M. Griffiths (2013), R. A. Davis (Davis 2001), A. Egorov, B. Johnson (Johnson 1999), P. E. Keck (Keck 2000), U. M.

Khosla (2000), Ts. Korolenko, D. J. Kuss (Kuss 2013), V. Laskutova, M. Lejoyeux (Lejoyeux 2010), S. Marks (Marks 2007), M. McMurran (McMurran 2004), E. Melnik, V. Mendelevich, J. Morahan-Martin (Morahan-Martin 2000), B. D. Ng (Ng 2005), M. Orzak, B. Segal, E. Usova, T. M. Schoenmakers (Schoenmakers 2013), N. A. Shapira N. A. (Shapira 2000), D. T. L. Shek (Shek 2016), G. W. Shorter (Shorter 2013), L. M. Shotton, A. Weinstein (Weinstein 2010), L. Widyanto (Widyanto 2004), P. Wiemer-Hastings (Wiemer-Hastings 2005), V. Yaroshevich, P. M. Yellowlees (Yellowlees 2007), K. Yang (Yang 2000), L. Yu (Yu 2016) and others.

The study of the issues of valuable and semantic sphere of students with Internet addiction is relevant, due to the fact that Internet addiction is becoming more and more widespread in adolescence.

The purpose of the work is to study the features of the system of valuable and semantic orientations of students with Internet addiction.

METHODS

Materials and Methods

Method of theoretical analysis of literature, comparison, synthesis of psychological information on the topic of research, test method, mathematical methods of statistics (R. Fischer's criterion).

Methods:

1. Test for determining Internet addiction by K. Yang (Yang 2000).
2. Test of life-sense orientations (the method of LSO) by D. A. Leont'ev (2000).
3. Method of determining the valuable orientations by M. Rokeach (Rokeach 2007).
4. Test "Diagnostics of real structure of valuable orientations of the personality" (Bubnova 2002).

The study was conducted at the Sevastopol State University. Fifty four undergraduate students of the 4th year study of technical specialty "Computer Science and Computer Engineering" took part in the research. It is important to note that all Young men were 20-23 years old.

An empirical study of the features of the system of valuable and semantic orientations of high school students with Internet addiction was conducted in several stages:

- The first stage is the selection of diagnostic research methods.
- The second stage is testing of diagnostic techniques.
- The third stage is processing the results of the study.
- The fourth stage is to check the statistical significance of differences in indicators.

At the first stage the theoretical and methodological basis of the research, problem, object, subject, hypothesis and tasks were determined in order to choose the research methods; theoretical analysis on the research problem.

At the second stage, the organization and conduct of research were carried out in order to identify the features of the valuable and semantic sphere in high school students with Internet addiction.

At the third and fourth stages, the data were systematized, analyzed, and interpreted.

Initially, K. Yang test was conducted to determine Internet addiction. (Yang 2000).

The test is a self-diagnostic tool for pathological Internet addiction (regardless of the form of this addiction).

Internet addiction is a phenomenon of behavioral addiction and emotional dependence on a particular form of behavior. From this point of view, addiction is characterized by three main symptoms:

1. Increasing the dose (time spent on the Internet increases)
2. Changing behavior patterns (Internet activity begins to replace real-life forms)

3. Withdrawal syndrome (deterioration of emotional well-being outside of Internet activity).

According to Kimberly Yang, the Internet additivity is determined by three main factors:

1. Availability of information, interactive zones, and pornographic images.
2. Personal control and anonymity of the transmitted information.
3. Internal feelings that subconsciously establish a greater level of trust in online communication.

The results are summarized in Figure 1.

The obtained esults indicate that 37.04% (20 people) of the respondents of the surveyed sample have Internet addiction. Internet addiction has not been detected in 46.29% (25 people) of the respondents, and 16.67% (9 people) of the respondents hasa tendency to Internet addiction. It should be noted that 6 people among the respondents with the identified tendency to Internet addiction have a weak trend. This indicator points out that it is possible to return quickly to the standart rate of Internet addiction using only willpower and Self control in the use of Internet resources. 2 people have a moderate tendency to develop Internet addiction, it requires more significant efforts to overcome this trend. 1 person has a high tendency to Internet addiction, it is possible to admit that it is almost formed. As well as identified Internet addiction, the high trend to Internet addiction requires serious corrective work.

It should be noted that we identified a large percentage of respondents of the surveyed sample with already formed Internet addiction, namely 46.29% (25 people) of the respondents. The obtained result obtained may be related to the specifics of the sample, namely, students of specialty "Computer Science and Computer Engineering." We assume that the passion for computer technologies and the Internet, as well as the professional significance of the computer and the Internet in particular, was the reason for such a high rate of Internet addiction among these students.

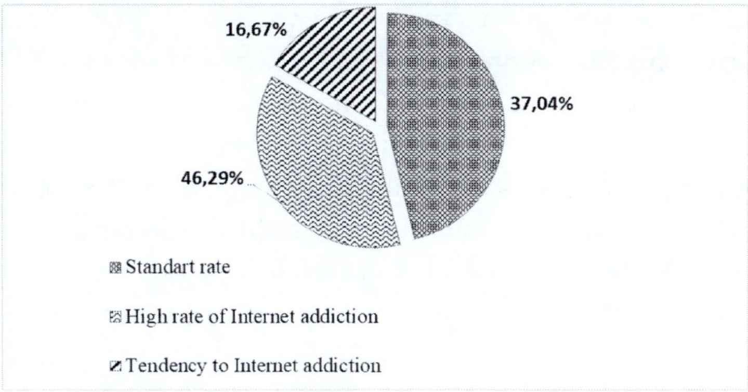

Figure 1. The indicator of Internet addiction among the respondents.

The test of lif'e-sense orientations by D. A. Leont'ev was conducted to determine the "source of the sense of living (Leont'ev 2000).

This method allows us to evaluate the "source" of the sense of living, which can be found by a person either in the future (goals), or in the present (process) or in the past (result), or in all three components of life.

The LSO test is an adapted version of "Purpose-in-Life Test" (PIL) by James C. Crumbaugh and Leonard T. Maholick. The method was developed on the basis of the theory of meaning and Logotherapy by Victor Frankl and aimed at empirically validating a number of representations of this theory.

The following subscales are used in the test: 1. The purpose of life. 2. The process of life or interest and emotional intensity of life 3. Effectiveness of lifestyle or satisfaction with self-realization. 4. The locus of self control (I am the master of life).

Method for determining the valuable orientations by M. Rokeach (Rokeach 2007).

M. Rokeach's test for the diagnosis of value orientation is one of the most popular questionnaires for the diagnosis of the valuable and semantic sphere of personality. This method allows you to explore the direction of the individual and determine his relationship to the world, to other people, to himself, the perception of the world, the key motives of actions, the basis of the "philosophy of life." M. Rokeach considered values as a kind of stable belief that a certain goal or way of existence is preferable to another. The nature of human values according to M. Rokeach: the total number of values that are the property of a person is relatively small, all people have the same values, although they are in different degrees, values are organized into systems, the origins of human values can be traced in culture, society and its institutions and personality, the influence of values can be traced in almost all social phenomena which are worthy of study.

The method developed by M. Rokeach is based on direct ranking of the list of values. M. Rokeach distinguishes two classes of values: terminal and instrumental. Graphically, the results are shown in Pictures 2 and 3.

The data obtained in the course of the diagnostic study using the method of D. A. Leont'ev's LSO (Leont'ev 2000) indicate that there are significantly more people with low and average indicators on the main scales of life-sense orientations in the group of respondents with identified Internet addiction and there are practically no high values, while in the group of respondents without Internet addiction, in most cases, prevail average and high values.

For example, the average indicator was found in 55.0% and low - in 45.0% according to "The goal in li" scale, in the group of students with Internet addiction, while in the group of students without Internet addiction, the average indicator was found in 91.18% and low – in 8.82%. This suggests that a significant part of students with Internet addiction tend to live for today or yesterday, and students without Internet addiction are characterized by the certain life orientations, purposefulness, orientation to the present and future.

According to "The process of life" and "The result of life scales," the group of respondents with Internet addiction also has a predominance of low (65.0%) and average (30.0%) indicators, while the group of respondents without Internet addiction has an average (91.18% - on "The process of life" scale and 73.53% - on "The result of life" scale) and high (5.88% – on "The process of life," 23.53% – on "The result of life") indicators. These results indicate a predominant dissatisfaction with their lives in the present and in the past in the group of students with Internet addiction.

According to “The locus self control” scale, both groups are dominated by average indicators (80.0% - students with Internet addiction, 70.94% - students without Internet addiction), which indicates an adequate assessment of their capabilities in building their own lives and implementing their plans. Some respondents with Internet addiction (15.0%) have a low indicator on this scale – this part of students does not believe in their own strength and the ability to control the events of their own lives, while the second group does not have such indicator, but 26.47% students have a high indicator on this scale – this part of students has an idea of themselves as strong personalities who have sufficient freedom of choice to build their life in accordance with their goals and objectives and ideas about its sense.

According to “The locus life-control” scale, only average and low indicators was found in both groups. Thus, in the group of students with Internet addiction, the average values was found in 75.0% and low - in 20.0%, while in the group of students without Internet addiction, the average values are 97.06% of the sample and low - 2.94%. This suggests that both groups of students are characterized by fatalism, the belief that human life is not subject to conscious control, that freedom is illusory, and it is pointless to think about something for the future.

Life-sense orientation of students with Internet addiction of the surveyed sample are characterized by the lack of significance for them such values as “The process of life”, “The result of life,” also “The purpose of life” is of less value. It can be concluded that students with Internet addiction are in the state of subjective sense of loss of meaning, which is a consequence of “existential frustration,” i.e., failure to find the meaning of life by a person. The absence of a goal in life colors it with a sense of meaninglessness of existence. The lack of satisfaction with your life in the present is associated with a weak emotional saturation of life. As a result, the result of the lived period of life does not bring satisfaction, all this in total leaves its mark on the perception of the prospects of life for the future.

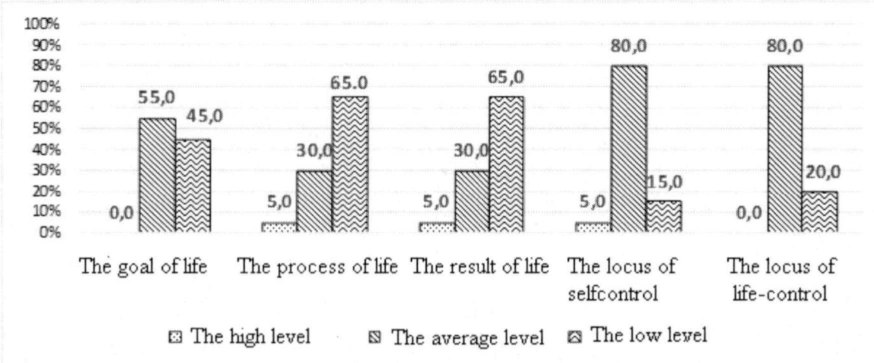

Figure 2. Generalized results based on the method of LSO by D. A. Leont'ev in respondents with identified Internet addiction.

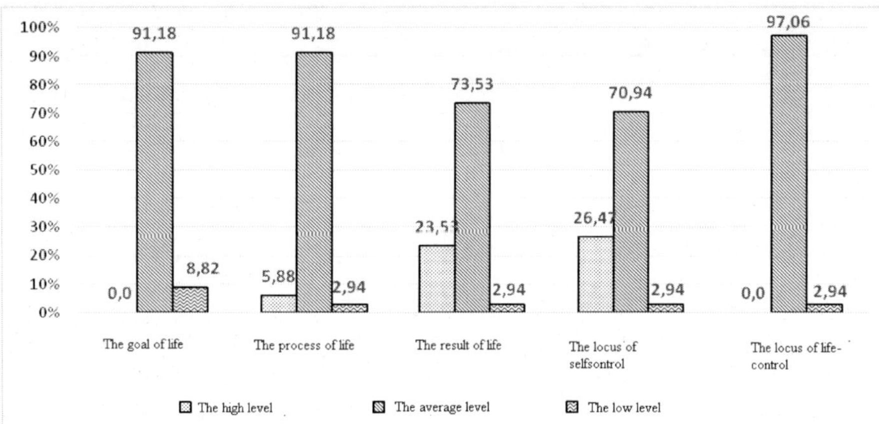

Figure 3. Generalized results based on the method of LSO by D. A. Leont'ev in respondents without Internet addiction.

The method by M. Rokeach was used to study the valuable orientations of respondents (Rokeach 2007). Graphically, the data is shown in Figures 4, 5, 6, and 7. The data obtained during the diagnostics show that respondents with and without Internet addiction have such terminal values of high importance as:

- having friends (students with Internet addiction - 85.0%, students without Internet addiction - 94.82%);

- family life (students with Internet addiction - 95.0%, students without Internet addiction - 88.24%);
- health (students with Internet addiction - 55.0%, students without Internet addiction - 94.82%).
- Less significant, but also important values such as:
- active life (students with Internet addiction - 65.0%, students without Internet addiction - 47.06%);
- productive life (students with Internet addiction – 60.0%, students without Internet addictionm- 44.12%);
- beauty (students with Internet addiction – 60.0%, students without Internet addiction - 44.12%).
- Insignificant values such as:
- development (students with Internet addiction - 50,0%, students without Internet addiction - 44,12%);
- happiness of others (students with Internet addiction - 75.0%, students without Internet addiction - 50.0%)

This distribution of values can be explained by the age characteristics of the sample. Student age coincides with the period of creating a family, choosing a profession, and active knowledge of the world.

An interesting fact is that for 90.0% of respondents with Internet addiction, love is a significantly important value, among listed above, while for 61.76% of respondents without Internet addiction, love was assigned to values of no sence. A fairly large percentage (50.0%) of respondents from both groups noted the importance of such value as wisdom. In the group of students with Internet addiction, the following values were not significant such as: work (60.0%), creativity (50.0%), confidence (55.0%), pleasure (65.0%), while in the group of students without Internet addiction, pleasure was marked as significant value (52.94%), and welfare (55.88%), knowledge (52.94%), freedom (52.94%) were not significant.

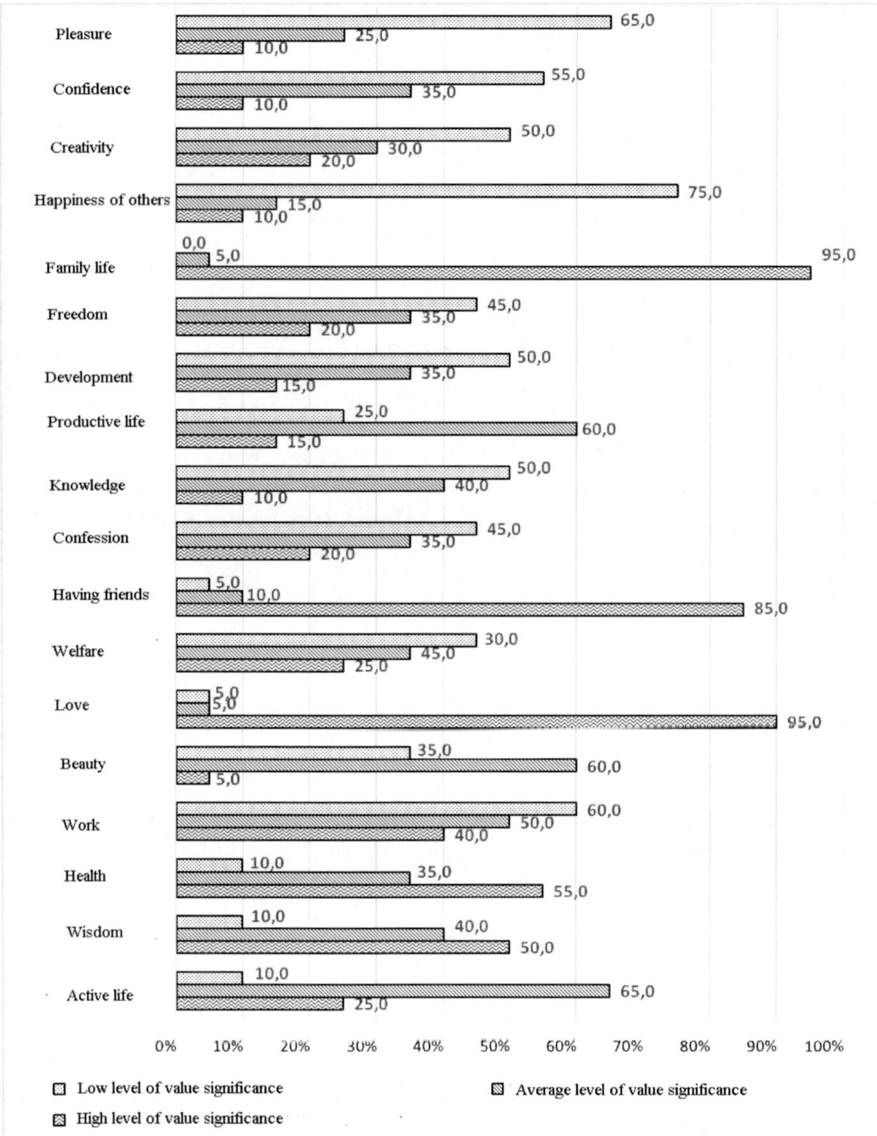

Figure 4. Generalized results of terminal valuesbased on the method by M. Rokeach in students with Internet addiction.

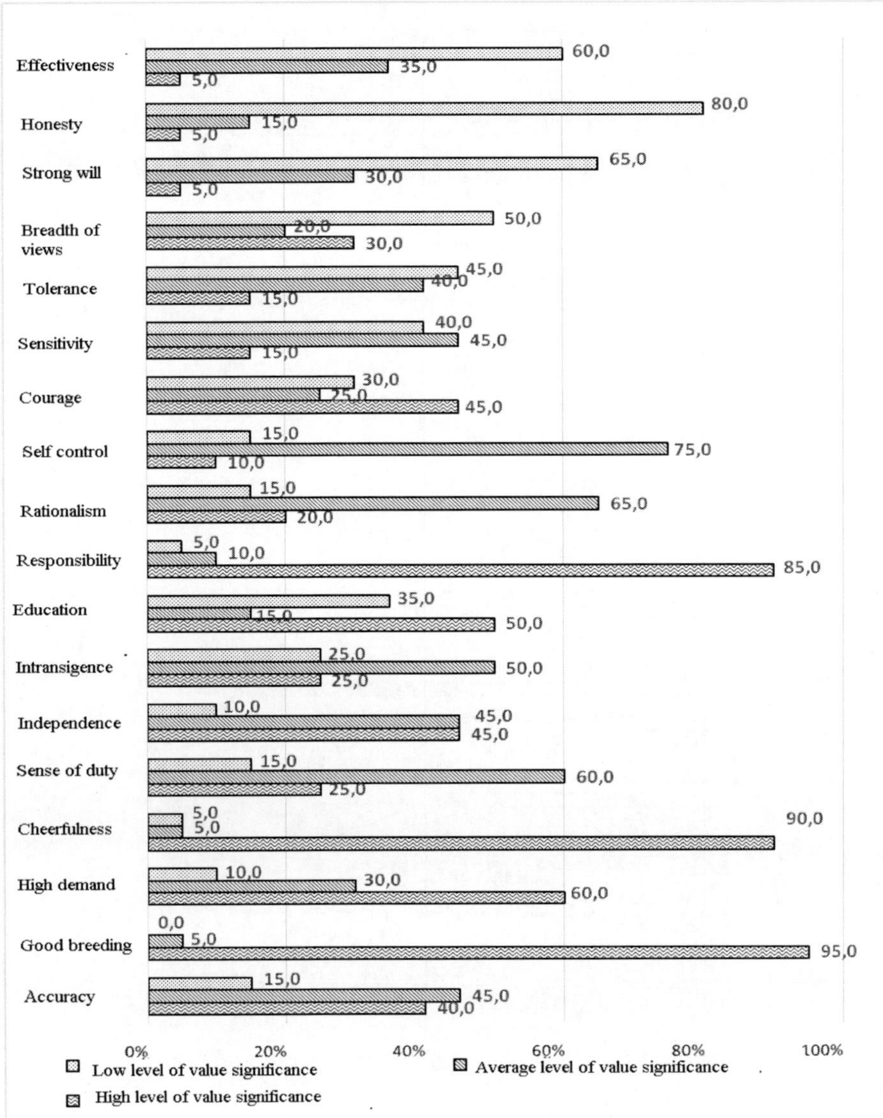

Figure 5. Generalized results of instrumental values based on the method by M. Rokeach in students with Internet addiction.

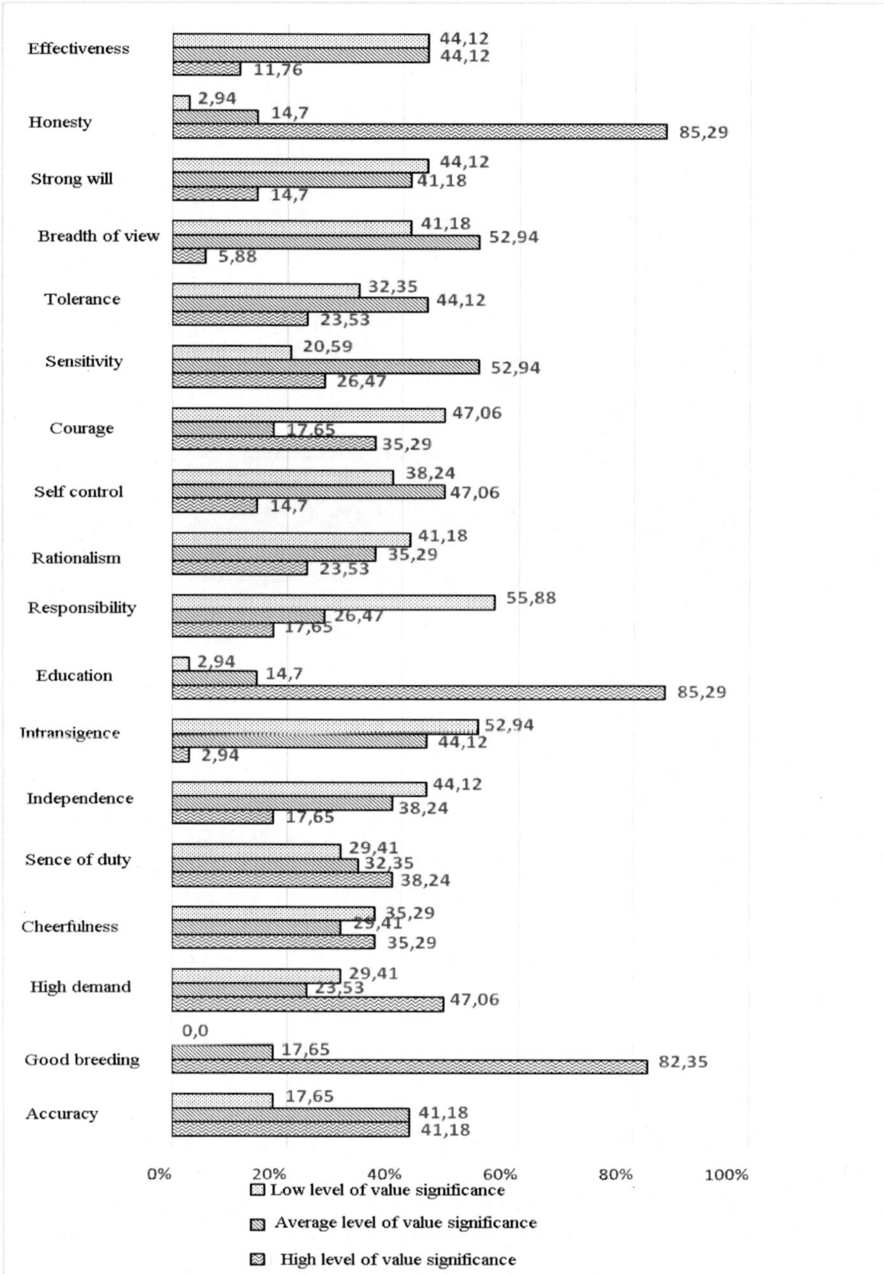

Figure 6. Generalized results of instrumental values based on the method by M. Rokeach in students without Internet addiction.

Among the instrumental values of both respondents with and without Internet addiction, good breeding is of high importance (students with Internet addiction - 95.0%, students without Internet addiction - 83.32%). The following values are also of high importance for respondents with Internet addiction: high demand (60.0%), cheerfulness (90.0%), responsibility (85.0%), courage (45.0%), accuracy (40.0%). And in the group of students without Internet addiction it is necssary to admit such instrumental values as honesty (85.29%) and education (85.29%) which are of high importance.

Self control is of a significant value for both groups of the sample (students with Internet addiction - 75.0%, students without Internet addiction - 47.06%). Students with Internet addiction also highlight rationalism (65.0%) and sence of duty (60.0%) among significant values, while students without Internet addiction - breadth of view (52.94%) and sensitivity (52.94%).

The following values are not significant for both groups of the sample: strong will (students with Internet addiction - 65.0%, students without Internet addiction - 44.12%), efficiency (students with Internet addiction - 60.0%, students without Internet addiction – 44.12%). For students with Internet addiction, such values as rationalism (65.0%), sence of duty (50.0%) are of little significance, and for students without it, responsibility (55.88%) and intransigence (44.12%).

Test “Diagnostics of real structure of valuable orientations of the personality” by S. S. Bubnova was also used to study the respondents' valuable orientations (Bubnova 2002). The method is aimed at studying the implementation of personal value orientations in real life conditions.

The author singles out the following values:

- Pleasant pastime, recreation.
- High material well-being.
- Search and enjoy the beauty.
- Help and charity to other people.
- Love.
- Learning new things in the world, nature, and man.

- High social status and people management.
- Recognition and respect of others influence them.
- Social activity to achieve positive changes in society.
- Communication.
- Health.

The generalized results for the sample are shown in Figures 7 and 8.

The obtained data as a result of diagnostics show that respondents with identified Internet addiction are more focused on pleasant pastime and recreation (expressed in 75.0%), love (expressed in 95.0%) than respondents without Internet addiction, who are more focused on achieving high material well-being (expressed in 82.34%), social status (expressed in 88.24%), recognition and respect for other people (expressed in 91.18%), the ability to manage and influence others, health (expressed in 82.35%).

Also, it should be noted that among respondents with Internet addiction, such values as: search and enjoy the beauty (55.0%), help and charity to other people (50.0%), recognition and respect for people and influence on others (70.0%), social activity to achieve positive changes in society (60.0%) are not expressed.

At approximately the same level, both respondents with and without Internet addiction expressed a desire to learn new things in the world, nature, and man (students with Internet addiction - 65.0%, students without Internet addiction – 82.34%), and focus on communication (students with Internet addiction - 90.0%, students without Internet addiction – 91.18%).

From the mentioned above, we can conclude that respondents with identified Internet addiction are more focused on hedonistic values (getting pleasure and enjoyment), while respondents without Internet addiction are more focused on socially significant values.

R. Fischer's f*-criterion was used to determine the statistical significance of the differences between the indicators of respondents with and without Internet addiction, using the method of LSO by D. A. Leont'ev, "Diagnostics of real structure of valuable orientations of the personality" by S. S. Bubnova and "Test for the diagnosis of value orientation" by M. Rokeach. An online calculator was used to calculate the value of f*-Fisher's criterion (Automatic Calculation of the Fisher Angular Conversion 2000).

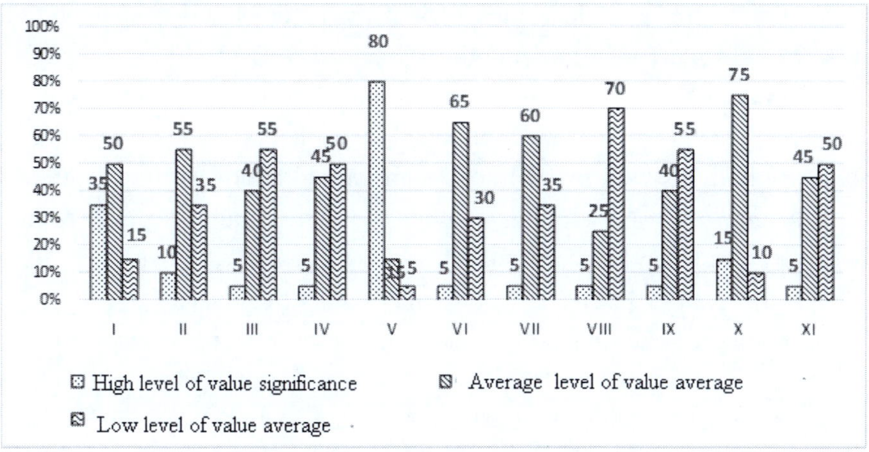

Figure 7. Generalized results based on the method of "Diagnostics of real structure of valuable orientations of the personality" by S. S. Bubnova in respondents with Internet addiction.

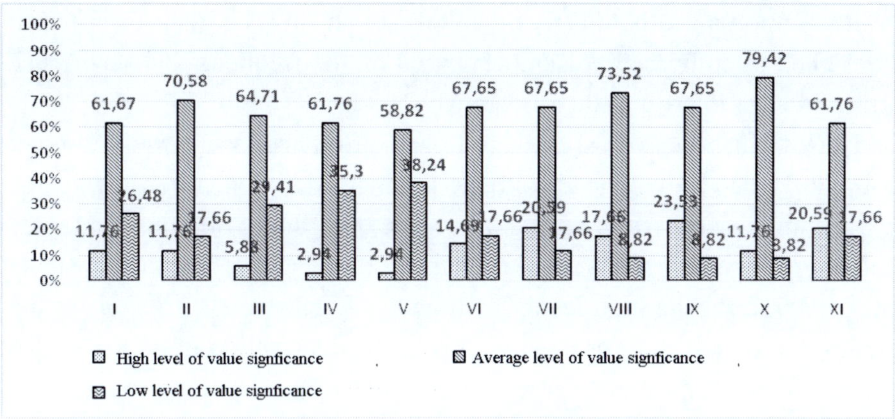

Figure 8. Generalized results based on the method of "Diagnostics of real structure of valuable orientations of the personality" by S. S. Bubnova in respondents without Internet addiction.

The results of the correlation analysis indicate that among respondents with and without Internet addiction, there are significant differences in such life-sence orientations as the goal in life, the process of life, and the result of life. Differences in values such as the locus of self control and the locus life-control are significant at the 1% error level.

The obtained data from the correlation analysis show that there are differences in the significance of such instrumental values as honesty among respondents with and without Internet addiction. At the 1% default level, differences were found in the following values: performance, cheerfulness, independence, intransigence, and breadth of views.

No significant differences were found on the other scales.

The results of the analysis indicate that among respondents with and without Internet addiction, there are no significant differences in the expression of such values as: pleasant time and recreation; high material well-being; help and charity to other people; knowledge of new things in the world, nature, and man; communication; search and enjoyment of beauty, high social status, and management of people. At the same time, there are significant differences in the expression of such values as love, recognition and respect for people and influence on others.

It is important to note Fisher's angular criterion. The Fisher's criterion is designed to compare two samples based on the frequency of occurrence of the effect of interest to the researcher.

During the research work, significant differences were found among groups of students with and without Internet addiction according to the Fisher's angular criterion: on the love scale, two diagnostic methods were used at once, namely the M. Rokeach method – f = 3.479 for the low level and f = 3.612 for the high level. S. Bubnova's method is f = 2.564 for the low level and f = 4.829 for the high level. The distribution of indicators for Internet addicts and non-Internet users is actually inversely proportional. M. Rokeach's method - students with an addiction of 18 people at a high level and 1 person at a low level to 5 people at a high level and 21 at a low level in students without addiction. S. Bubnova's method - with an addiction of 16 people at a high level and 1 at a low level to 1 at a high level and 13 at a low level in students without addiction. This allows us to conclude that love is an extremely significant value for those suffering from Internet addiction. The need for love is one of the most urgent age-related needs of the youth period. The emergence of love is a response to a certain need, and it initially manifests itself in the form of feelings. The need itself is not obvious, it is hidden in the depths of the unconscious, and it is the feelings that connect it with consciousness. And if the non-dependent student has these feelings directed at an object from real life, then the Internet addict redirects it to the virtual. On online pages, they meet, communicate, fall in love with their virtual interlocutor, creating an invented, illusory image of their beloved, with the hope of meeting in real life. Such correspondence can last for weeks, months, and the desired meeting may not happen. In turn, the average Young man by this age already has a certain social experience in the field of communication, Dating, tactile contact with the opposite sex. For him, the process of falling in love (communication, kissing, sex) is not something extra-ordinary, unusual, significant, which can be highlighted in the first place in his life. Thus, due to the age-related need for love and the difficulties and obstacles of translating virtual love into real life, the Internet-dependent Young man identifies this value as one of the most significant.

There was also a difference in the statistical results of the respondents on the honesty scale according to the method of M. Rokeach, $f = 4.982$ at the high level and $f = 4.141$ at the low level. The results are inversely proportional, in addicts 1 person has high level and 18 has low one, 28 has high level and 1 has low one in independents. These indicators tell us that honesty is not a significant value for online addicts. Communication on the Internet is famous for its ability to remain completely anonymous. A user who is afraid of public speaking can freely Express themselves and defend their point of view in comments and forums without fear of public condemnation. Being honest is not practical in a place where you can't check how much information about you is valid.

In addition to honesty, there is difference in the scale of recognition and respect for people and the influence of others according to the method of S. Bubnova $f = 3.481$ at the low level, $f = 2.046$ at the middle level, and $f = 1.624$ at the high level. Among the addicts, 11 people are on low level,

8 on average one, and 1 on high level, while other students have 3 on low level, 25 - on average one, and 6 - on high. One of the features of the Internet that attracts users so much is the ability to become a different person, which the gaming industry has especially had a hand in. Every year there are various military simulators, strategies, role-playing games that allow you to try yourself in role of a hero of the Second world war, a professional motorcycle racer, a special forces soldier, a knight, and even a God. At the same time, since 2012, competitive elements, various leaderboards, special privileges for successful cyber fighters, weekly clan battles, and others have been actively introduced into games. All these factors allow you to achieve respect not for real people around you-friends, relatives, classmates, but to show the level of self-aggrandizement among the same players, to self-actualization with the help of virtual success. The motivation to build social connections and status disappears quickly if success and recognition can be achieved in the game field, even if it is virtual.

CONCLUSION

In the surveyed sample of 54 students, Internet addiction was detected in 37.04% (20 people) of respondents. The tendency to Internet addiction is observed in 16.67% (9 people) of respondents. The high level of Internet addiction is conected with the peculiarities of the chosen specialty.

According to the method of LSO by D. A. Leont'ev, it was revealed that a significant part of students with Internet addiction tend to live for today or yesterday, they are mostly dissatisfied with their lives in the present and in the past. Students without Internet addiction are characterized by the presence of certain life orientations, purposefulness, orientation to the present and future. In both groups of respondents, an adequate assessment of their capabilities in building their own lives and implementing their plans was found, but 15.0% of students with Internet addiction do not believe in their own strength and the ability to control the events of their lives. It was also revealed that both groups of students are characterized by fatalism, the belief that a person's life is not subject to conscious control.

According to the method of M. Rokeach, such values as having friends, family life, and health are of high importance among the terminal values, both for respondents with identified Internet addiction and without it. Such values as an active and productive life, and beauty are less important, but also important. Values such as development and the happiness of others are not important. Among the instrumental values education is of high importance for both groups of respondents as with as without Internet addiction.

According to the method "Diagnostics of real structure of valuable orientations of the personality" by S. S. Bubnova respondents with identified Internet addiction are more focused on pleasant pastime and recreation than respondents without Internet addiction, who are more focused on achieving high material well-being, social status, recognition and respect for other people, and the ability to manage and influence others. Among respondents with Internet addiction, such values as search and enjoyment of beauty, help and charity to other people, recognition and respect for people and influence on others, social activity to achieve positive changes in society are almost not expressed.

The results of the correlation analysis indicate that significant differences in the expression of such values as love, recognition and respect for people and influence on others, and honesty were found among respondents with and without Internet addiction. The high importance of love for addicts is associated with the inability to fully implement virtual love in real life. Differences on the 'honesty' scale are related to the fact that an online user can always remain anonymous on the network and express any thoughts without fear of punishment, and also post false or inaccurate information about themselves. Differences in the scale of recognition and respect for people and the influence of others are associated with the possibility of self-realization in the cyber space.

REFERENCES

Automatic Calculation of the Fisher Angular Conversion 2000; URL: https://www.psychol-ok.ru/statistics/fisher/.

Bubnova S. S. 2002. *Diagnostics of the Real Structure of Personal Value Orientations*; URL: http://hr-portal.ru/tool/metodika-diagnostika-realnoy-struktury-cennostnyh-orientaciy-lichnosti-ss-bubnova.

Davis R. A. 2001. Cognitive-behavioral model of pathological Internet use. *Computers in Human Behavior.* No 17(2), pp. 187–195. URL: https://doi.org/10.1016/S0747-5632(00)00041-8.

Johnson B. 1999. Three perspectives on addiction. *Journal of the American Psychoanalytic Association.* https://doi.org/10.1177/00030651990470031301.

Kuss D. J., Shorter G. W., M. D. Griffiths, Schoenmakers T. M. 2013. Internet addiction components model. *International Journal of Mental Health and Addiction*, No 11(5), 1–26. https://doi.org/10.1007/s11469-013-9459-9.

Leont'ev D. A. 2000. *Test of Life Orientations*; URL: https://psycabi.net/testy/256-test-smyslozhiznennye-orientatsii-metodika-szho-d-a-leontev.

Morahan-Martin J., & Schumacher 2000. Incidence and correlates of pathological internet use among college students. *Computers in Human Behavior*, No 16(1), No 13–29. https://doi.org/10.1016/S0747-5632(99)00049-7.

Ng B. D., & Wiemer-Hastings, P. (2005). Addiction to the Internet and online gaming. *Cyberpsychology and Behavior*, 8(2), 110–113. https://doi.org/10.1089/cpb.2005.8.110.

Rokeach M. 2007. *The Nature of Human Values*; URL: https://studfiles.net/preview/1711139/.

Shapira N. A., Goldsmith T. D., Keck P. E., Khosla U. M. & McElroy S. L. 2000. Psychiatric features of individuals with problematic internet use. *Journal of Affective Disorders*, No 57(1–3), 267–272. https://doi.org/10.1016/S0165-0327(99)00107-X.

Shek D. T. L., Yu L. & Sun R. C. F. 2016. *Internet addiction. Neuroscience in the 21st Century: From Basic to Clinical, Second Edition* pp. 3707–3750. Springer New York; URL: https://doi.org/10.1007/978-1-4939-3474-4_108.

Weinstein A., & Lejoyeux M. 2010. August. Internet addiction or excessive internet use. *American Journal of Drug and Alcohol Abuse*. https://doi.org/10.3109/00952990.2010.491880.

Widyanto L., & McMurran M. 2004. The psychometric properties of the internet addiction test. *Cyberpsychology and Behavior*, 7(4), 443–450. https://doi.org/10.1089/cpb.2004.7.443.

Yellowlees P. M., & Marks S. 2007. Problematic Internet use or Internet addiction? *Computers in Human Behavior*, 23(3), 1447–1453. https://doi.org/10.1016/j.chb.2005.05.004.

Young K. 2000. Diagnoz – Internet-Addiction. *Mir Internet*. No 2. P. 24–29.

In: Psychological Service … ISBN: 978-1-53618-160-9
Editor: Svitlana V. Kucherenko

Chapter 8

DIRECTIONS OF THE UNIVERSITY PSYCHOLOGICAL SERVICE' WORK: IN-DEPTH PSYCHOLOGICAL DIAGNOSTICS OF THE 1ST YEAR STUDENTS AS A FACTOR OF LEARNING EFFICIENCY IN HIGHER EDUCATION

Marianna A. Latysheva*[*]*, PhD
and Eugene Y. Brunner*[†]*, PhD
Psychology Department,
V. I. Vernadsky Crimean Federal University, Crimea, Russia

ABSTRACT

The article deals with the importance of functioning of university psychological service for the first-year students, targeting psychological

[*] Corresponding Author's Email: maralat@yandex.ru.
[†] Corresponding Author's Email: brunner_eu@mail.ru.

diagnostics in particular. The need for conducting an in-depth psychological diagnostics for contemporary first-year students is theoretically proved, a possible battery of psychodiagnostic methods is put forward. It is assumed that psychodiagnostic results present the optimal starting point for designing a student's individual educational route, for monitoring his/her professional and personal development during the course of study.

Keywords: university psychological service, psychological diagnostics, first-year students, individual educational route, professional and personal development

INTRODUCTION

The problems of organizing the psychological service in the higher education system have been in the field of view of domestic researchers for decades (Abulhanova-Slavskaya 1993; Kolosov, Bobylev and Kruchinin 2007). Recent years show a clear need for psychological support of the professional formation of a future specialist due to several reasons. On the one hand, the demands for a student expertise, level of personality development "output" increase and on the other, many students appear not to be ready to solve many tasks put before them by the educational environment of the university and by the specific age phases. In particular, in the modern practice of higher education institutions, the volume of independent work of students, the number of creative and problem tasks, the obligation to participate in project and research activities, etc. increases every year. At the same time, for the majority, student life is the first experience of living a relatively independent life, the need to make decisions themselves, to build a new system of relationships, etc. The above reasons, both collectively and individually, can destabilize the psycho-emotional state of students, provoke the development of stress, depending on what ground they appear.

Thus, in order to preserve the psychological health of future specialists the question of how to optimize the psychological support of students at the stage of mastering the profession remains relevant for the psychological service of the university.

In this regard, the purpose of this article is to justify the need for mandatory for the 1st year students in-depth psychological diagnostics focused on building a system of support taking into account long-range planning of their personal and professional development, as well as multi-subject design of conditions necessary to achieve it (in the case of Psychology students).

METHODS

Participants

Over the past decade, the psychological service has become an integral part of the educational system. The role of psychological support for the educational process in higher education has also increased, the importance of which is actively discussed at different levels by representatives of the Ministry of education, in the framework of scientific and practical conferences, in scientific publications. It should be clearly stated that in the conditions of modernization of the system of higher professional education (HPE) the implementation of the tasks facing the HPE becomes rather difficult without qualified psychological support for the process of training specialists in various fields.

The university psychological service is a structural specialized division that prioritizes the personal and professional development of students and carries out its activities in accordance with the principles of humanization of education and a personality-oriented approach (Kaltaeva 2011).

Modern problems of development and organization of the university psychological service, analysis of working experience and various models of implementation of psychological assistance in individual universities are covered in a number of works (I. E. Lilienthal, C. B. Nedbayeva, N. G. Shcherbanyova, E. I. Metelkova, Yu. V. Sukhoveyshina, V. V. Zhidkova, N. V. Volodko, M. V. Kaltaeva, etc.) (Volodko 2010; Zhydkova 2006;

Kaltaeva 2011; Liliental 2000; Metelkova 2010; Nedbaev and Zhidkova 2003; Shcherbaneva 2003). It should be noted that the psychological service in education is a practical tool that adapts scientific psychological knowledge to the immediate needs of employees in the field of education and at the same time allows one to identify urgent and possible problems in this area.

Prospects for the development of psychological services in higher education institutions are determined by basic target areas. Among them there are such as increasing the opportunities of the educational environment of a university in the development of personal and professional competence of its graduates, improving the effectiveness of interaction between the subjects of the pedagogical process, building a system of functioning of psychological services of educational structures at different levels (complete general education-intermediate professional education-HPE), of a university and of partner enterprises, for example, enterprises where specialized university departments function. Grounding on the works of such domestic scientists as A. G. Asmolov, I. B. Kotova, A. B. Petrovsky, V. A. Petrovsky, V. I. Slobodchikov, E. N. Shiyanov, etc., as well as on the practical experience of our university we can state that adaptation and personality development at the stage of mastering the profession are components of a single process of personality socialization.

The organization and functioning of the university psychological service is regulated by the following principles: the principle of democratization of higher education, the humanization principle, the principle of individual activity, the principle of ethical and psycho-hygienic norms; the principle of the unity of scientific, applied and practical aspects of its activities in the university; the principle of ensuring the implementation of diagnostic, prognostic and management functions to all the university and higher education system subjects; the principle of ensuring the leading role of the university in the entire system of continuing education, in the economic and cultural life of a region (Efremova 2015; Kolosov, Bobylev and Kruchinin 2007; Ozhygova 2015; Pahal'yan 2003; Pilyugina and Berezhnova 2012; Umnyashova and Mkarova 2017).

In recent years, psychological services have been established in a number of Russian universities, which operate on the basis of various models.

Among the most common options for organizational models and psychological services M. Bityanova names the following: the model of student psychological service, the model of "psychological assistance study," the model of psychological support for the personal development of students, the model of psychological support for the educational process at the university and the model of psychological support for managerial processes at the university (Bityanova 2010). At the same time, the choice of a particular model is determined by the personnel capabilities and professional position of the specialists of certain university, the requests and position of the university administration, the material and technical conditions of the psychological service, etc.

It is obvious that in the process of studying at a university, students inevitably have difficulties or even serious problems that are specific to different stages of their education. A number of empirical studies have shown that students in various fields of training not only need psychological help, but also note to some extent the importance and necessity of psychological knowledge in their life (Kojchueva 2005). So, among first-year students, the primary difficulty is the very process of studying at a university, the need to establish interpersonal relationships in the group and adaptation to new educational demands and conditions. In the second and third years, as a rule, educational motivation decreases, frustration and doubts arise as to the adequacy of the choice of profession, problems of practical application of existing knowledge emerge, etc. Students of the fourth year of study are usually concerned about understanding their own achievements in professional development and the need to determine the further professional path, the search for a job. Such issues as increasing self-confidence, developing public speaking skills, developing interpersonal relationships, and developing communication, leadership, and organizational skills are also relevant. In other words, the above-described problems of students of different years of study to some extent affect their psycho-emotional state, results and quality of their activities, including the effectiveness of their training.

Thus, our colleagues' research on the main psychological problems of students at different stages of professional training allows us to talk more reasonably about the need to build a system of psychological support for students, covering all stages of professionalization, starting with the career guidance stage (pre-university stage), and ending with the vocational selection stage (graduation courses).

It is known that currently the main activities of the psychological service are psychological education, psychological diagnostics, psychological prevention, psychological correction, research activities, organizational and methodological activities, psychological construction, psychological examination (Dubrovina 1998).

We will limit ourselves with the focus on one of the areas of psychological service activity, namely, on the psychological diagnostics. In our opinion, currently the university needs to review the opportunities of applying psychological diagnostics. This is due to significant changes in the state of the modern youth population and to the inadequacy of a solely psychometric approach when assessing the mental state of young people studying, to increasing innovation in education and focusing on the individual educational route of a student, and in our region, to such an aspect as the multi-ethnicity of students. In this regard, providing effective psychological support to students at all stages of their professional training, in our opinion, requires an *in-depth psychodiagnostic examination* in order to obtain a qualitative assessment of the characteristics of a student's mental state and development, starting from the moment of his/her admission to the University.

The term "in-depth psychological diagnostics" was introduced by N. Semago and M. Semago and reveals the specifics of the psychologist's diagnostic work during individual examination of children and teenagers (Semago and Semago 2016). At the same time, the authors suggest not a usual testing, but namely a psychological evaluation, which is understood as the collection and integration of data obtained using such methods as observation, clinical interview, clinically oriented research methods, including psychological tests, etc. It should be noted that the authors, on the basis of their extended professional experience, offer a modern three-component model for analyzing the mental and somatic state of modern children, which forms the bedrock for a new typology of development, including the deviant one.

The proposed model is based on the idea of the basic structural organization of psyche as a process (Figure 1) (Semago and Semago 2016).

As you can see, these levels are vertically organized and consist of the causal, basic structural organization of psyche as a process and phenomenological levels. On the basis of the proposed model, it becomes possible to analyze the key moments of changes (transformations) of mental development systematically, implementing into practice the idea of "non-disjunction" of mental formations into "natural" and "higher" ones. For example, the evaluation of the neurobiological component of development as a relatively independent component of the causes of the observed features of the child's mental development provides an understanding of its compensatory capabilities, and hence the accuracy of the prognosis.

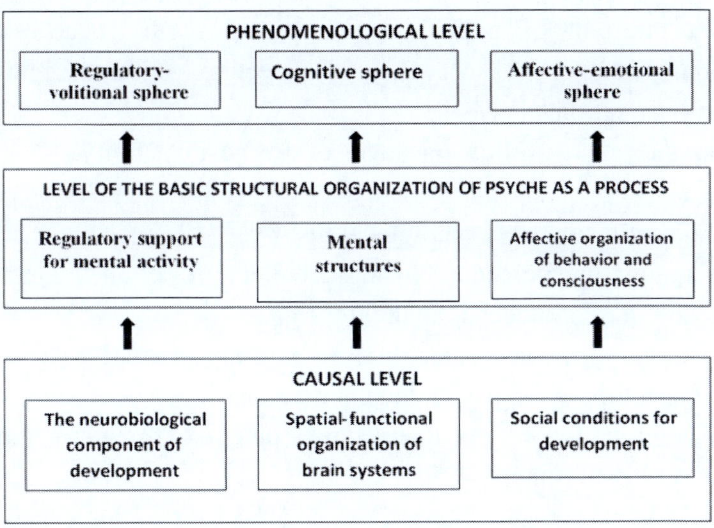

Figure 1. Three-component model of mental development analysis, by N. Semago and M. Semago (N. Semago and M. Semago 2016).

"The central element ... of the analysis is the" basic structural organization of psyche as a process "," which ".. manifests itself in the individual originality of behavior, cognitive styles and strategies of activity, in personal characteristics and in the nature of relationships with the surrounding world" (Semago and Semago 2016, 49).

Obviously, qualitative changes in the development of the system of basic components can be found in other critical moments of a person's growing up, one of which is his/her "entry" into the profession, primarily at the stage of acquiring HPE.

In this regard, we consider it possible and necessary to use the term "in-depth psychological diagnostics," as well as a three-component model and, with certain refinements, also the description of the stages and the survey procedure itself, in order to reach the goal we set.

The technology of the in-depth diagnostic activity presupposes the need to identify certain stages, which will allow one to carry out within the university system a comprehensive assessment of the current mental state of a first-year student, his personal characteristics, i.e., to describe the psychological diagnosis and on its basis to formulate a reliable prediction of his further development and training. These data can be directly used to develop a program of individual educational route, if necessary, to determine the ways of the most effective corrective work at the initial stage of professionalization.

So, we suggest the following stages of diagnostic activity:

1. The collection of psychological history.
2. Examination procedure (using a battery of certain recommended techniques and questionnaires)
3. A comprehensive system analysis of the examination results and a description of the psychological diagnosis
4. Determination of the likely development expectation, individual educational route.

We will briefly describe each stage.

The first stage presupposes conducting a structured interview – collecting the student's psychological history. In accordance with the general principles of psychological diagnostics, the history of human development, or anamnesis, is the source of building a psychological diagnostic hypothesis. In the framework of the proposed form of examination, a psychological history, which reflects the family and social situation of the student's development in different age periods, is important. Thanks to this, we obtain data on the existence of acute or chronic injuries, the type of family education, and .etc. during periods of key transformations of the student's mental development, which may be in a latent state and may manifest in the adaptive period.

At the *stage* of the *examination* itself, we suggest using the following psychodiagnostic battery: Individual-typological questionnaire (ITQ, by L. N. Sobchik), "Level of personal subjectivity development" technique (LPSD, by M. A. Shchukina); colour attitude test (CAT, by M. A. Etkind); "Recognition of idioms and metaphors" technique (by T. V. Chernigovskaya, V. L. Deglin); E. Kraepelin's counting test (Golovey and Ribalko 2002; Egorov 2006; Semago and Semago 2016; Sobchik 2013; Shchukina 2014).

Such a selection of psychodiagnostic techniques provides an opportunity to evaluate within a short period of time the features of the formation of the basic components of the student's mental development (voluntary regulation of mental activity; cognitive, affective and emotional sphere), his individual psychological profile. In particular, multiannual research conducted by L. N. Sobchik convincingly showed that leading trends (according to the author, a leading trend includes the conditions for a certain trait of personality forming as well as the trait itself and the predisposition to the state which can be developed under the environmental influences and become the continuation for the said trait) shape the constitution and character of the individual, determine the basic parameters of his life – interests, social activity, choice of profession, life partner.

The level of personal subjectivity development technique (LPSD, by M. A. Shchukina) is used to identify the level of development of personal subjectivity and the structure of non-situational personal subjectivity, i.e., the ability that provides a person with the opportunity to exercise self-government in the social context of their being. The level of formation of personality subjectivity in a first-year student gives clarity in understanding how able he/she is to independently manage his life in its various manifestations, in which directions and in what form this student can be assisted at the training stage (by professors, a university psychologist, administration).

The color attitude test (CAT, by M. A. Etkind) will allow us to evaluate the features of the student's attitude to a number of significant concepts (such as future profession, most/least favourite academic disciplines, professional prospects, professional attitudes, etc.), as well as the range of significant persons, including those from the faculty. By assessing the emotional components of a student's personality relationships, we can quickly find the "hottest spots" in the system of his/her relationships and minimize their consequences, because often they are either not realized or deliberately hidden by the subject.

The "Recognition of idioms and metaphors" technique (by T. V. Chernigovskaya, V. L. Deglin) is used to rapidly evaluate the role of the left and right hemispheres in the speech and mental activity of a student, his/her tendency to addictive behavior. This data allows us to clarify the cognitive style, the specifics of information processing, the reasons for difficulties in mastering the material, etc. in a particular student.

E. Kraepelin's counting test estimates the level of a student's mental performance and fatigue, the rate of his/her mental activity and satiety. Operational characteristics of activity are extremely important indicators of the human mental productivity as a whole. As one of the integrative characteristics, it reflects the pace changes with the change of motivation, the level of self-regulation in a student's activity.

The stage of a comprehensive systemic analysis of the survey results determines specific individual characteristics of each student's development and gives a sufficient description of the specific structure of his mental activity and personality (psychological diagnosis).

The final stage presupposes making a prognosis of the student's development, taking into account his/her potential and adaptive capabilities in the educational space, and, consequently, developing an individual educational route for the period of mastering the profession.

It is known that the predicting mechanism includes a systematic analysis of the psychological characteristics of the student's personality, identifying the actual development needs, the zones of actual and expected development, the peculiarities of the social environment and interpersonal relationships, in accordance with which the development tasks at this stage of ontogenesis are determined, an individual development trajectory is developed, taking into account all subjects of the psychological and pedagogical space, and a description of the necessary conditions for its implementation. This stage becomes the starting point for monitoring the professional and personal development of the student throughout the entire period of study and involves the appropriate adjustment of previously set goals and objectives. The experience of the implementation of qualified psychological and pedagogical prediction of the students development has shown the importance of organizing the professional interaction of teachers and psychologists on the basis of the psychodidactic principle.

Thus, the technology of in-depth diagnostic activities carried out by the university psychological service from the initial stage of professional training provides each of the students with the opportunity to build prospects for the near future, both personal and professional, based on individual characteristics, interests, health conditions and educational environment. It should be noted that such providing of students with psychological support, psychological knowledge and skills forms in students a positive life attitude, a strategy of life path, in which getting a profession, career development, and achieving success in life are viewed as important milestones. Thus, from the first year of studying students develop meaningful responsible behavior.

In this regard, the responsible position of other participants in the educational process is also important. We mean the university administration, the teaching staff, whose activities should provide a favorable psychological atmosphere within the university.

Here it seems essential to describe the specifics of other activities of the psychological service that are closely related to the in-depth psycho-diagnostics of the first-year students. Familiarization with its results is carried out within the framework of psychological counseling, which, taking into account the tasks set, is aimed at 3 subjects of education – students, the teaching staff, and the university administration.

Counseling students is focused on offering them the results of psychological diagnostics, which integrate individual student data, general tasks of age group and patterns of professional development. The main goal is to motivate the student to build a promising model of his/her own professional and personal growth, to create in him/her the desire to develop an individual educational route together with teachers. Obviously, this amount of work involves several meetings.

Consulting the teaching staff allows us to present in a generalized systematized way the results of an in-depth psycho-diagnostics of the entire group of first-year students and to highlight the most important recommendations for building relationships with individual students, teaching didactics, and the formation of the design and construction activities of a teacher (Lyaudis 2008). In particular, in one of the empirical studies devoted to the investigation of individual psychological patterns of personality of psychology students, the characteristics of their cognitive style are described, which allows teachers to adjust their classroom performance, select tasks for independent work and perform differentiated control of knowledge testing (Latysheva 2016). Thus, socially passive individualists and rigid students better absorb systematic material and freely operate digital information presented in the form of symbols, schemes. At the same time, students with conformal, dependent personality traits are focused primarily on the verbal way of mastering information. Emotionally labile and anxious students also well absorb new material in a verbal form, but in combination with bright sensory images.

Consulting the university administration is focused on presenting the generalized results of the in-depth psycho-diagnostics of a group of first-year students, explication of promising tasks for this student group according to the stages of their professional training.

Another type of activity of the psychological service is psychological correction. In our opinion, psychological correction of first-year students can be differentiated as to the following directions. The first is aimed at students with low adaptive potential, or identified signs of maladaptation. The second includes a group of first-year students whose individual and personal characteristics are in the zone of pointed accentuated traits, and disagree with the requirements of the profession. The third direction is aimed at students with an insufficient level of formation of the basic components of mental development (voluntary regulation of mental activity; cognitive, affective and emotional sphere).

Within the framework of psychological education, taking into account the peculiarities of the Crimea, a number of lectures on the following topics will be held for first-year students:

1. Psychological readiness to create an educational route.
2. Development of gender identity and opportunities for men and women in the family and profession
3. Directions of innovative activity of youth in the Crimean region
4. Prospects for intercultural cooperation in a multi-ethnic region.

According to our forecast, the final result of the activities of the psychological service of the Humanitarian and Pedagogical Academy, the Tauride Academy aiming at the implementation of the technology of in-depth psychological diagnostics of first-year students majoring in 37.03.01. "Psychology," will be like that – optimization of the process of adaptation to the educational environment of the university, increase in educational motivation; responsible behavior relating to the development of professionally important personality traits, conscious formation of an individual style of professional activity, professional identity, a positive life attitude of a future specialist.

CONCLUSION

Individual psychological and personality characteristics of first-year students can become an obstacle to the successful mastering the profession.

To solve the problems of modernizing the system of higher professional education, improving the quality of professional training of specialists in various fields, including psychologists, it is necessary to use the potential of university psychological service.

In particular, the suggested technology of in-depth diagnostic activity is focused on a comprehensive assessment of the level of basic components of mental development, personal characteristics of first-year students and prediction of its further development and studying at the university. Individual results are the basis for the development of the program of a student's individual educational route, which can significantly improve the quality of training, as well as update students' responsibility for their own life.

The described system of mutually reinforcing types of practical activities, such as in-depth psychological diagnostics, psychological correction, psychological education, unfolding within the framework of the psychological service, provides a meaningful integration of all the subjects of education - students, the teaching staff and administration of the university.

Thus, the activities of the university psychological service make it possible to provide psychological and pedagogical conditions contributing to the development of the personality of a future specialist in the field of psychology, who is motivated to live up to his/her potential, is socially and psychologically stable, and effectively adapts to changes in the professional sphere and public life.

Of course, the proposed solution to the problems of modern education is only one of the possible solutions and requires empirical verification and support from the university administration.

ACKNOWLEDGMENT

The authors of the article express their deep gratitude to all the participants of the experiment.

REFERENCES

Abulhanova-Slavskaya, K. A. 1993. "Tipologiya lichnosty i nekotorye zadachi psychologicheskoy sluzhby v vuze. [Typology of personality and some tasks of psychological service at a university.]." In *Psychologicheskaya sluzhba v vuze: printsipy, opyt raboty*, edited by B. B. Kossov, 33-43. Moscow. (In Russian).

Bityanova, M., and Beglova, T. 2010. "Modeli deyatelnosti psichologa v obrazovatelnom uchrezhdenii. [Models of psychologist's activity at the education institution.]" *Shkolnyj psicholog* 2:23-27. (In Russian).

Dubrovina, I .V. 1998. "Psychologicheskaya sluzhba obrazovaniya : nauchnye osnovaniya ,tseli i sredstva. [Psychological education center: scientific grounds, goals and means.]." *Psychologicheskaya naucha i obrazovanie* 2:5-9. (In Russian).

Egorov, A .U. 2006. *Neyropsichologiya deviantnogo povedeniya.* [*Neuropsychology of Deviant Behavior.*]. Saint-Petersburg: Rech. (In Russian).

Efremova, O. I. 2015. "Psychologicheskaya sluzhba vuza kak odin iz institutov professionalizatsii budushchih psichologov obrazovaniya. [University psychological center as one of the institutions of professionalization of future educational psychologists.]" *Vestnik Taganrogskogo institute im. A. P. Chehova* 2: 257-262. (In Russian).

Golovey, L. A., and Ribalko, E.F., editor. 2002. *Praktikum po vozrastnoy psichologii.* [*Workshop of a developmental psychology*]. Saint-Petersburg: Rech. (In Russian).

Kaltaeva, M. V. 2011. "*Teoreticheskie I organizatsionnye stanovleniya i razvitiya psychologicheskoy sluzhby vuza.* [*Theoretical and organizational foundations of the formation and development of the psychological center of the university.*]" PhD diss., Nizhnegor.gos. architect.-stroit. University. (In Russian).

Kolosov, E. V., Bobylev, V. N., and Kruchinin, V. A. 2007. "Psychologicheskaya sluzhba vuza: teoriya i praktika. [University counseling center: Theory and Practice.]" *Vysshee obrazovaniy v Rossii* 3:10-13. (In Russian).

Kojchueva, F. H. 2005. "*Psychologicheskoe soprovozhdenie lichnostno-professionalmogo razvitiya studentov yuridicheskogo fakulteta*. [*Psychological support for the personal and professional development of law department students*.]" PhD diss., Stavropol. (In Russian).

Latysheva, M. A. 2016. "Kontseptualnye osnovy psichologicheskogo obespecheniya obrazovatelnogo protsessa v sisteme vysshego obrazovaniya. [Professional training of future psychologists with various individual psychological personality patterns as a psychological and pedagogical problem.]" In *Conceptualnie osnovi psihologicheskogo obespecheniya obrazovatelnogo processa v sisteme gumanitarnogo obrazovaniya: kollektivnaya monografiya*. 374–394. Ufa: AETERNA. (In Russian).

Liliental, I. E., 2000. "*Psychologicheskaya podderzhka studentov v period adaptatsii k obrazovatelnomu protsessu*. [*Psychological support of students in the period of adaptation to the educational process of the university*.]" PhD diss., Stavropol. (In Russian).

Lyaudis, V. Ya. 2008. *Metodika prepodavaniya psichologii*. [*Psychology teaching methods*.]. Saint-Petersburg: Piter. (In Russian).

Metelkova, E. I. 2010. "Psychologicheskaya sluzhba kak resurs razvitiya sovremennogo obrazovaniya. [*Counseling center as a resource for the development of modern education*]" PhD diss., Mosk.gor. psichol.-ped. University of Lobachevskogo. (In Russian).

Nedbaev, S. V., and Zhidkova, V. V. 2003. "Psychologicheskaya sluzhba vuza. [University counseling center.]" *Psychologiya v vuze* 3:49-59. (In Russian).

Ozhygova, L. N. 2015. "Psychologicheskaya sluzhba v vuze: nauchnye i prikladnye zadachi soprovozhdeniya professionalnogo obucheniya. [University counseling center: scientific and applied tasks of vocational training support.]" *Razvitie sovremennogo obrazovaniya: teoriya, metodika I praktika* 3 (5):88-91. (In Russian).

Pahal'yan, V. E. 2003. *Psihoprofilaktika v prakticheskoj psihologii obrazovaniya*. [*Psychological prevention at the practical psychology of education*.]. Moskow: PER SE. (In Russian).

Pilyugina, E. I., and Berezhnova, O. V. 2012. "Psychologicheskoe soprovozhdenie lichnostno-professionalnogo razvitiya studenta vuza. [Psychological support of personal and professional development of a student.]" *Molodoy uchenyj* 10:289-291. https://moluch.ru/archive/45/5480/. Accessed February 01, 2020. (In Russian).

Semago, N. Ya. and Semago, M. M. 2016. *Teoriya i praktika uglublonnoyi psikhologycheskoyi diagnostiki. Ot rannego do podrostkovogo vozrasta.* [*Theory and practice of in-depth individual psychological diagnostics. From early age to teenagers.*]. Moskow: ARKTI. (In Russian).

Shcherbaneva, N. G. 2003. "*Psychologicheskaya poderzhka professionalnogo razvitiya studentov pedagogicheskogo vuza sredstvami psychologicheskoj sluzhby.*" [*Psychological support for the professional development of students of a pedagogical university by means of a university counseling center*]. PhD diss., Armavir. (In Russian).

Shchukina, M. A. 2004. "*Osobennosti razvitiya sub'ektnosti lichnosti v podrostkovom vozraste.*" [*Peculiarities in personality subjectivity development in teenagers.*]. PhD diss., Tumen. (In Russian).

Sobchik, L. N. 2013. *Individualno-tipologicheskiy oprosnik . Ppракticheskoe rukovodstvo k tradicionnomu i komputernomu variantam testa.* [*Individual-typological questionnaire. Practical guide to the traditional and computer-based test forms.*]. Moskow: Kompaniya BORGES. (In Russian).

Umnyashova, I. B., and Mkarova, I. V., editor. "*Psychologicheskaya sluzhba University: realnost i perspektivy.*" [*University counseling center: reality and prospects.*]. Materialy I Vserossiyaskoj nauchno-prakticheskoj konferencii s mezhdunarodnym uchastiem, Moskow: FBGOUVOMUPPU NIU VSHE. 27-28 oktyabrya 2017. (In Russian).

Volodko, N. V. 2010. "*Psychologicheskie usloviya organizatsii psychologo-pedagogicheskogo prostranstva tsentra detskogo razvitiya.* [*Psychological conditions for the organization of the psychological and pedagogical space of the center for child development.*]" PhD diss., University of Lobachevskogo. (In Russian).

Zhydkova, V. V. 2006. "*Razvitie psychologicheskoy sluzhby pedagogicheskogo vuza*. [*The development of the psychological service of a pedagogical university.*]" PhD diss., Kursk. (In Russian).

In: Psychological Service …
Editor: Svitlana V. Kucherenko
ISBN: 978-1-53618-160-9

Chapter 9

Directions of the University Psychological Service' Work: Psychological Counseling as the Basis of Applied Psychologists' Activity

Inobat A. Erina*[*], *PhD
Psychology Department,
V.I. Vernadsky Crimean Federal University, Crimea, Russia

Abstract

The article deals with the problem of Crimeans seeking opportunities for further self-determination in mainland Russia. Presented is a theoretical overview of various scientists' opinions concerning the field of students' pedagogical integration. Discussed is the importance of practical psychologists' assistance needed by students from the very beginning of their studies. Considered are the theoretical foundations of

[*]Corresponding Author's Email: irinagorbushina@mail.ru.

counseling. The article provides an in-depth analysis of the forms of psychological counseling as the basis of practical psychologists' activity. Identified are the problems and tasks of psychological counseling.

The present research into the problem has allowed identifying three typical reasons for conducting psychological counseling and singling out the stages of the psychological counseling process. Considered are the methods used by psychologists in the counseling process. Presented is the code of psychological consultants' professional ethics which regulates their professional activity.

Keywords: practical psychologist, psychological counseling, integration, students, forms, methods, stages, psychological counseling code

INTRODUCTION

The system of education in the Russian Federation has recently focused attention on students' integration throughout the country. Nowadays, students are given an opportunity to choose opportunities of their career development at various universities located not only in their hometowns but also in other regions. The criteria for the high quality of Russian education are currently based not only on the processes of learning and acquiring new knowledge, but are also closely related to practice.

In this regard, the relevance of psychological counseling as the basis of practical psychologists' activity is increasing.

METHODS

Participants

On the one hand, people's life has recently become more interesting. However, it tends to cause more difficulties. Nowadays, people face a number of problems in their life trying either to avoid them or solve them on their own.

Unfortunately, the decisions people take not always help them to cope with complex problems in their life.

Facing problems they cannot solve on their own, most people try to circumvent them, forget about them, postpone their solution or, under certain circumstances, give in. Sometimes people find solutions which may lead to various predicaments in the future: at the social level, interrelationship with relatives, colleagues, etc. may be handicapped, while at the psychological level, a person may acquire various phobias, panic attacks, depressed states, feeling of guilt, apathy, aggression, etc. As a rule, one needs to seek help from a psychological counselor in such a situation.

Thanks to the Crimea's reunification with Russia, young people choosing their future professions can consider the educational institutions of the peninsula; and the Crimeans residing in Russia's mainland have an advanced opportunity of their personal identity formation. Such students' integration into the student community presents a certain degree of coincidence and similarity in opinion, orientation, etc. in relation to the whole student group. As for the educational aspect of life, the integration process affects the interconnections of all participants of the educational and extracurricular processes. The interaction and the interrelationship within a group are some of the main aspects of the group's activity.

S. Y. Golovin (2001) believes that integration should be considered a process occurring within a group, manifested by the developing unity of its goals and guidelines as well as team-work. As a result of interaction, the group members will have to represent a single entity, where everyone can hedge and support the others, be responsible for the successes and failures in the group's joint activities.

According to L. M. Shipitsina (2001) integration is a one-way process divided into the social and pedagogical types. She believes that social integration affects only the individual's adaptation processes within the environment he or she is integrated into (e.g., the educational environment).

Pedagogical integration, in its turn, should affect and shape the individual's abilities, which will facilitate his or her integration in the future.

Analyzing the scientific research on the given problem, it is necessary to consider integration as a bidirectional process in which not only individuals adapt to the community, but also the community adapts to them.

Nowadays, higher education institutions train professionals in various fields, and young people's choice is not always based on their abilities and desires. Most likely, their choice is a budgetary state institution where they can study for free.

On entering higher education institutions, they immediately face the difficulties connected with mastering the fundamentals of their would-be professions.

Applied psychologists can help in this situation giving professional advice. The society has developed various attitudes towards such specialists. While some people cannot live without them and seek their advice on every minor occasion, others go to such specialists only when they are deadlocked and do not know what to do next, and still others feel strongly that it is a waste of money and no one can help them.

Such attitudes are generated by people's ignorance as to the essence of psychological counselors' professional activity. Such specialists neither give advice nor provide ready-made blueprints for resolving their clients' problems. Advising their clients, psychological counselors provide expert opinions on the problems and touch upon the internal resources and possibilities of the client's deep potential based on his or her own experience. Moreover, they provide their clients with a range of possible solutions so that the clients could choose the most satisfactory way out of the tight corner.

The main and most important point in counseling is that clients should feel responsible for their actions taken after counseling in order to make changes in their life.

In the psychological encyclopedia, psychological counseling is presented as a form of providing practical psychological assistance in the form of advice and recommendations given on the basis of preliminary research into a client's personality and his or her problems, as well as the client's relationship with other people (Bubnova S. 2000).

There are various definitions of psychological counseling.

American psychotherapeutic counselors believe that counseling is a special kind of assistance relationship, its efficiency depending on the good client - counselor relationship facilitating positive changes in the client's life. Burks and Steffir believe that psychological counseling is a qualified consultant's professional relationship with his or her client, which is usually characterized by an individual approach, although sometimes more than two people are involved in it.

E. E. Sapagova (2001) believes that psychological counseling is a form of professional psychologists' activity, which consists in direct interaction with people with the aim of helping, making decisions regarding the circumstances and conditions of their personal and social life, aimed at achieving psychological comfort, personal growth and change in behavior.

According to Y. B. Alyoshina, psychological counseling consists in direct interaction with people aimed at solving various kinds of psychological problems associated with difficulties in interpersonal relations, where the main method of influence is a certain type of conversation. Psychological counseling has various definitions in scholarly literature (Alyoshina Y. 2003).

A. N. Elizarov (2001) notes that "it is an applied branch of modern psychology. Within the framework of psychological science, its task is to develop theoretical foundations and applied programs for providing psychological assistance to mentally and physically healthy people in situations when they face psychological problems. These theoretical foundations and programs are developed on the basis of an analysis of the current state of psychological research and achievements in the fields of empirical and theoretical research".

Thus, psychological counseling is an integral part of individual and group psychological assistance to various categories of clients. This type of psychological assistance is closely connected with other forms of active influence on someone's personality, such as psychological correction, psychotherapy, etc. The specific character of this method consists in direct bilateral focused communication between the counselor and the client, usually in the form of a confidential individual conversation.

Counseling is intended to provide psychological assistance to healthy people experiencing various difficulties in real-life situations in order to solve their problems. The psychotherapeutic intervention is aimed at solving in-depth personal problems underlying the majority of real-life difficulties and conflicts.

The benefits of psychological counseling include:

- comparative simplicity,
- profitability,
- ability to provide immediate emergency assistance.

A significant number of clients live under acute or chronic stressful conditions, experience difficulties in social adaptation, have unstable social motivation and difficulties in interpersonal relationship or suffer from deviant behavior. Besides, they experience difficulties at critical age periods requiring psychological support and correction aimed at solving their problems. Therefore, psychological counseling needs objective professional consideration and further development in social care services. Practicing psychologists are advised to choose this type of psychological assistance.

Analyzing the basic principles underlying the theory of counseling allows determining the important principle of understanding the continuous process of life-long socialization and personality development. It was put forward and substantiated in humanistic psychology and psychotherapy by Carl Rogers and Erik Erikson. This approach suggests that the process of personal growth continues or resumes even in difficult situations which seem inextricable. Each person has sufficient internal resources to overcome the problems of psychological growth and development delay, as well as an internal development potential, which is independent of external living conditions.

In addition to the continuous process of life-long socialization and personality development, one can mention the concept of sensitive and crisis periods of personality development. This concept is presented in Eric Erickson's scholarly works. R. Nelson-Jones believes that psychological counseling, in its essence, is a type of assistance relationship (Burmenskay G. 2002).

In her methodological guidelines, N. V. Klyueva presents the basic concepts of consulting psychology and characterizes psychological counseling. She pays much attention to the professional competencies and personal characteristics of psychological counselors, as well as the requirements imposed on them. Tracing back the history of this form of rendering assistance services, it can be said that people turned to shamans, priests and even magicians with their problems from time immemorial. The very first counselors were Moses, Lao Tzu, Buddha, Confucius, Socrates, Plato and Aristotle who were healers, philosophers and clergymen. Hippocrates, the forefather of psychological counseling, considered it essential to create the atmosphere of trust while treating people asking for help in order to more accurately understand and determine the particular characteristics of their diseases. His first classification of mental disorders and the definition of the term "temperament" are still used nowadays (Klyueva N. 2011).

The 19th century marked a special stage in the development of psychological counseling. Practical psychology as a science appeared when the first scientific experimental laboratory was established by W. Wundt in Germany. The outstanding discoveries in the treatment of hysteria made by S. Freud and J. Breuer proved to be the basis of medical counseling in psychiatry. Medical assistance began with the use of medications, and then psychotherapists also provided their assistance.

The rapid changes taking place in the society encouraged the scientific community to search for new forms of psychological assistance and specialists who would provide them. In the mid-1940's, psychological counselors were mainly engaged in diagnosing their clients' individual characteristics while dealing with various problems, for example, difficulties in communication, interaction and the emotional sphere.

Thanks to Carl Rogers, the rapid development of this type of assistance began in the 1950's and the 1960's. His client-centered therapy became the theoretical basis for training psychological counselors. Carl Rogers's book, "Counseling and Psychotherapy" (1942), provided new scope for psychological counseling. From that year on, this branch of psychological knowledge began to separate from the related branches (psychiatry, psychotherapy, etc.). Earlier, psychological counseling was considered within the framework of medicine, so psychological counselors were mainly engaged in detecting their clients' individual characteristics, focusing exclusively on vocational counseling (mainly vocational counseling at school).

The 20th century witnessed intensive development of psychological counseling, especially vocational counseling. The overwhelming majority of such specialists (80 percent) were trained to work at secondary schools holding vocational counseling.

Carl Rogers (Rogers 1957) insisted that people having difficulties in communication and interaction are not mentally ill (previously such clients were mainly treated by psychiatrists and psychotherapists), so most of them do not need medical treatment. Providing them with support is the main way of getting rid of their difficulties. Within the framework of the humanistic trend, 7 stages of the counseling process are distinguished:

1. Defining whether internal communication is blocked internally. It is expressed in the lack of desire to change and the denial of the problem.
2. Self-expression. At this stage, the client reveals his or her feelings and problems.
3. The progress in the self-disclosure process.
4. Admitting one's own difficulties, inconsistencies and restrictions.
5. Classifying one's phenomenological world. Accepting one's inner world. "Become yourself".
6. Developing congruency. Integrating one's personal experience into a unity.
7. Personality changes. Opening up to oneself and the surrounding world.

The main techniques of the humanistic trend are as follows:

1. Reflective listening.
2. Mirroring.
3. Metaphors and intuition.
4. Repetitions (retelling).
5. Generalization.
6. Empathic responses.

At about the same period of time, various branches of psychology spread and developed widely, such as gestalt therapy, transactional analysis, behavioral counseling, etc.

Each trend competed with the others, making a certain contribution and delivering benefits.

In order to build effective patient - counselor relationship, R. Carcuff (2001) and his colleagues developed the methods of evaluating psychological counselors' efficiency, relying on the systematic approach and focusing on the development of their professional skills.

In 1929, the first counseling center providing psychological assistance on marriage and family matters was opened in New York.

In the 1930's, particular attention in the United States was drawn to the development of strategies of psychological counseling in the field of employment. Under E. Williamson's guidance, the first theory of "trait factor" counseling was developed at the University of Minnesota.

In Russian practical psychology, there are several approaches to understanding the essence of psychological counseling.

Present-day psychological counseling is based on the principles inherited from earlier stages of its development, namely:

- searching for an answer to vital questions, it is impossible to find the absolute truth or the only possible way out;
- numerous alternatives and opportunities can be proposed to try and solve a problem (Burmenskay G. 2002).

According to N. N. Obozova (2002) psychological counselors should, first and foremost, clarify the causes and consequences of real-life situations, and not offer new behavior profiles. In her opinion, psychological counselors' main task is to provide their clients with professional assistance so that the clients should be able to put their problems into perspective and discuss all the aspects of their relationship which seem to cause problems, but are usually not recognized and not controlled.

A. F. Kopieva (2002) believes that the "dialogical breakthrough" is an important stage in counseling, presenting the culmination point of the counseling process, when the client's painful isolation is overcome in relation to the essential aspects of his or her life.

According to V. D. Mendelevich, psychological counseling is the analysis of clients' mental state with the help of interviewing, experimental psychological research yielding objective data and scientific interpretations of the results. These are supposed to facilitate solving clients' psychological problems, introducing new ideas about various approaches to their prevention, solution and methods of psychological defense and compensation, as well as improving clients' psychological culture and encouraging their personal growth.

Taking into account the above-mentioned reasoning and making an intermediate conclusion, it can be argued that the main form of impact in counseling is changes in clients' attitudes.

Counseling gives a client an opportunity to look at situation from different perspectives, evaluate his role in it and, as a result, adjust his behavior patterns and attitude to what has happened.

It seems fair to say that psychological counseling is one of the main types of psychological assistance a person can be provided with. Its main purpose is to provide results-oriented professional psychological assistance.

Leading scientists and starting psychotherapists, as well as practical psychologists resort to this kind of assistance in their practical activities. Having mastered it, they can more highly qualified in treating their clients. Covering the topic of the article presupposes answering the question "Why is this type of assistance considered to be the main one in psychologists' professional activity?"

The possible answers are as follows:

1. Counseling helps clients to realize their role in particular problem situations.
2. Counseling helps to choose the solution to the problem for which the client will take up responsibility himself.
3. Counseling emphasizes clients' independence and positive client - counselor interaction.
4. Counseling provides an opportunity to develop one's personality and helps clients to acquire new behavior patterns.
5. Counseling is oriented not only towards individual clients, but also groups, communities, etc.

Thus, psychological counseling is a type of psychological assistance affecting not only clients' personal aspects, but also their status in the society.

Nowadays, psychological services are becoming relevant in overcoming difficult real-life situations. The ongoing changes in the society affect the psychological aspect of people's life. Even during the peacetime of the 21st century, people are faced with local wars, a large number of refugees and internally displaced persons, as well as an increase in the number of natural disasters, personal tragedies, and family life difficulties. People have to experiences any kinds of difficulties in resolving these situations, so they need timely psychological assistance. Unfortunately, not all people understand its essence and the ways such psychological assistance is provided. What tools does a psychologist work with?

In human life, words are of paramount importance (the way they are pronounced, what points are stressed in speech, etc.).

In the beginning was the Word, thus begins the first line of the Gospel of John (the New Testament). Cyril and Methodius translated the Greek concept of Logos by the concept of the Word. In philosophy, "logos" is the word carrying an inseparable thought.

Poems have been written about words. In 1956, the Russian poet Vadim Shefner wrote the verse "Words" in which there are the following lines: "One can kill with a word, one can save with a word, one can lead regiments with a word".

Psychological counseling also makes use of words and their collocations. Bearing the above-mentioned information in mind, one can say that Psychological counselors need to be knowledgeable not only of the assistance methods and techniques, but also the ability to conduct a dialogue with both a client and a group of clients.

At present, psychological counseling is a service provided by various counseling centers and private psychological counselors. Nowadays, the job position of a psychologist is considered a good investment in different organizations, since the profession of the "man-man system" is really counted on.

Psychological counseling is usually conducted in the form of a conversation, hence the concept "counseling conversation". Revealing this concept as the main form of psychological counseling, it is necessary to emphasize that it is a process of dialogic communication in which a person (counselor) helps another one (client) to use his or her internal resources for personal development in a positive direction.

As it has been mentioned above, this kind of assistance can be offered only to individuals but also to groups of people.

In this regard, one can distinguish the following kinds of counseling:

- intimate and personal (individual counseling),
- family counseling,
- pedagogical counseling,
- business counseling.

All these kinds are closely related, as they share common features. Nevertheless, they differ in certain specific features, such as activity management.

As for providing clients with counseling, psychological counselors need to take into account particular clients' individual typological properties constituting the knowledge base of the given counseling case.

The society consists of various social groups consisting of people. These groups are divided into the following classes:

- demographic (women, men, children, elderly people, young people);
- ethno-social;
- socio-economic (poor, rich, middle class people);
- professional;
- people with special educational needs.

Seeking psychological assistance, people want to solve different kinds of problems. Therefore, psychological counselors' qualification training is of great importance. At present, higher education institutions and institutions of further education train such specialists both in Russia and abroad. A number of psychological disciplines are included in the curriculum of such programs: developmental psychology, ethno-psychology, social psychology, family psychology, etc.

It is impossible to provide professional psychological counseling if one is unaware of the essence of personality and group development or the psychological mechanisms underlying particular difficulties. A very important aspect of professional development is self-education (participation in trainings, joint practical exercises, etc.), which allows to acquire a number of professional skills.

In the process of psychological counseling, it is necessary to have such skills as active listening, reformulating statements, explanation, generalization, ability to ask questions, interpretation of events, reflection of feelings, provision of support, empathy and information, exposure ability, etc.

A counselor's personality is essential for counseling effectiveness. While interacting with clients, counselors share their life and professional experience, values and worldview attitudes.

The object of psychological counseling comprises the following problems:

1. Difficulties of age development.
2. Features of adaptation to the changing features of everyday life.
3. Personal relationship disharmony (including not only family relationship, but also intimate, child-parent, peer relationship, etc.).
4. Social disabilities, e.g., drug addiction, alcoholism, sexually transmitted diseases, etc.
5. Various consequences after a serious illness, injury or stress.
6. Individual character traits.
7. Career choice and development.
8. Psychological and personality development.

For psychological counselors it is essential to make sure that clients choose solutions to their problems independently.

Before starting the psychological counseling process, it is necessary to determine its format and the tasks to be addressed.

The choice of tasks can be different and depends on clients' requests.

According to R. S. Nemov, counselors should address the following tasks during the psychological counseling process:

1. Naming the problem.
2. Defining the gist of the problem and its severity level.
3. Measuring the resource potential of the client's personality.
4. Formulating numerous recommendations.
5. Providing ongoing assistance when the client is already solving the problem.
6. Training the client to prevent problems in the future.
7. Providing the client with basic psychological knowledge and skills.

B. D. Karvasarsky distinguishes the following tasks of psychological counseling:

1. Emotional support and attention to the client's experience.
2. Extension of knowledge and increase of psychological competence.
3. Change in attitude to the problem.
4. Increasing stress resistance and crisis tolerance.
5. Developing a realistic and pluralistic worldview.
6. Increasing responsibility and developing readiness for the creative development of the surrounding reality.

When is it necessary to provide psychological counseling? What steps should it include?

An analysis of the scientific and practical literature has revealed three typical reasons for conducting psychological counseling:

1. The client seeks help; this situation is considered the most favorable one, since initially he is ready for effective interaction with the counselor.
2. The client is invited to a consultation. Most often it happens to clients registered with social welfare bodies and families experiencing difficulties when psychological counseling is necessary to relieve possible psychological stress and anxiety.
3 The client is advised to consult a psychologist by his or her bosses or management. As a rule, present-day organizations employ professional psychologists who work directly and indirectly with the staff in general and with each staff-member in order to solve various problems (stress relief, settlement of conflict situations, etc.). This process is fraught with difficulties, since psychologists act as intermediaries between the management and the staff; the counseling process may be blocked by clients.

In the counseling process, psychologists need to rely on the basic personality theories (paradigms): psychoanalysis, behaviorism, existential, cognitive, gestalt, interactive theories and ethical personal idealism.

Now we shall proceed to psychological counseling's stages.

According to A. Abramova, the structure of the counseling process is more understandable, since it implies asking questions, and the counseling process is divided into several stages at which the above-mentioned researcher offers particular questions, for example (Abramova A. 2005).

- "What is the problem?";
- "What do you want to achieve?";
- "What else can be done?";

"Are you really going to do it?"

At the preparatory stage, the counselor takes the client's case history and his or her problems. The obtained information helps to select suitable methods for further assistance.

The main stage presents a natural continuous process of controlled and guided patient – counselor interaction. Its obligatory elements smoothly follow each other and include the basic techniques of psychological counseling:

1. Asking Questions

Open or closed questions are used at the initial stage of counseling. Using this technique, psychological counselors encourage their clients to talk out, add or reword their statements. The technique also provides an opportunity to illustrate one's problems with examples.

2. Encouragement and Reassurance

The technique is used to create and strengthen the direct patient – counselor contact. It also includes non-verbal methods of communication (nodding, knowing look, etc.).

3. Rephrasing

The technique shows the client that great attention is being paid to what he or she is saying. At this stage, it is important to articulate the client's main idea.

4. Generalization

The technique helps to single out the main idea of several statements which are not closely related to each other. It provides an opportunity to stimulate discussion of significant topics in the future.

5. Reflection of Feelings

The technique implies focusing on the subjective aspects, confessions, statements, and trying to understand them.

6. Silence Technique

It has 2 types:

- meaningful,
- meaningless.

It can occur as a signal symptom of insight, or in a case of resistance.

7. Providing Information

The technique consists in expressing well-grounded opinions in response to clients' questions.

8. Psychological Interpretation

The technique implies explanation of the client's words. It consists in making an "assumption of something" with such words as "perhaps", "supposing", "probably".

9. Confrontation

It is used to show the psychological defenses that the client uses, thus limiting his or her development in order to draw the client's attention to contradictions in behavior, thoughts or feelings. Besides, the technique can be applied when the client shies away from discussing some problems. It must not be used to destroy psychological defenses.

10. Self-Disclosure

The technique helps to strengthen credibility with clients and is used as a reaction to the matter discussion (here and now).

The methods used by psychologists in the counseling process will be considered below.

Psychodiagnostic testing can be considered the main and traditional method. It allows to get qualitative and quantitative indicators about one's mental processes, conditions and properties. It is advisable to use it when it is not possible to establish the true cause of the problem in a conversation. Projective techniques and methods of positive psychology are most commonly used in psychodiagnostic testing.

Dynamic observation. In the counseling process, psychologists need to monitor their clients' reactions, conditions and personality characteristics. In this case, psychologists act as experts and can purposefully model problem situations in a conversation. They should pay attention to verbal means of communication, non-verbal reactions, autonomic manifestations, etc. Such observation should go unnoticed by clients.

Emotional charging. It consists in purposeful direct transference of psychologists' positive feelings to their clients in order to correct their mental state and form the most favorable psychic atmosphere contributing to the best possible relationship between the psychologist and the client. The specific feature of this method is that psychologists must control their emotions.

Suggestion. It is a direct verbal impact on clients' mental state in order to change their opinions, attitudes and behavior. Suggestion should be used to remove psychological defenses and overcome clients' direct resistance in a conversation. The method is optional and should be applied only in case all the other attempts at influencing a person have failed.

Persuasion. This method enables counselors to prove the arguments and reasons logically conveyed against the background of a person's balanced emotional state. It is considered to have a mild though noticeable influence on the client's psyche because it helps to correctly understand and interpret what the client said, find common ground with him and promote further communication.

An important role in psychological counseling is played by the conditions of its implementation. It is advisable to conduct it in a room designed specifically for this purpose. The "feel at home" environment of trust in this room will favorably influence both the process and the result of counseling. The counselor must take into account the counselor – client distance, the position of his arms and legs during the counseling process, as this can stress out the client. It is advisable to maintain eye contact during the counseling process. Psychological consultations should not be too long at a time. Moreover, they should be based on the ethical principles of psychological counseling.

Counselors take up responsibility and have obligations to their clients, the institution or company they work at, their colleagues and the society in general. In this regard, every country has adopted its professional code of conduct regulating psychological counselors' professional activity. The main points of these codes are as follows:

1. Privacy. It has 2 levels: the limit of professional use of clients' information and the conditions under which the information may be used.

   The circumstances in which the principle of privacy may be violated are as follows:

   - Increased hazards to the client's or other people's life
   - Criminal acts such as violence, incest, sexual abuse of children
   - The need for the client's admission to hospital
   - The client's or other people's involvement in a crime
   - The client is put on notice of the need for more effective assistance, provided by specialized services, social assistance services.
2. Counselors are strongly advised not to consult their relatives, friends, students or sexual partners.
3. Friendly and unconditional acceptance. Counselors should accept their clients as such. It is impractical to impose the same requirements on all clients and give the same recommendations to them. In order to make the counseling process effective, is

necessary to take personal factors and circumstances into account. It should be made clear to clients that counselors are not indifferent. On the contrary, they want to understand their clients and evaluate their possibilities and abilities objectively.

4. Clients' rights for making independent decisions at any stages of the counseling process should be respected. Clients' rights are respected as human rights to determine their fate, lifestyles and patterns of life, have their own convictions, opinions and views of life. To start with, psychological counselors determine not only their clients' problems, but also their needs, possible ways of solving their problems and the expected final results of the counseling process.
5. Personal responsibility.
   Developing a joint action plan with their clients, psychological counselors look into not only the essence of the clients' problems, but also about their needs. Psychological counselors are responsible for the quality of the assistance they provide, thoughtfulness and accuracy, as well as for the atmosphere of acceptance, openness and creativity allowing for deep positive changes in their clients' perception.
6. Respect for clients' rational expectations.
   The "do not harm" principle is followed in stabilization and harmonization of clients' interaction in the society.

In conclusion, it should be emphasized that nowadays it is necessary to spread information about professional practical psychologists, involving them in the psychological follow-up of Crimean students' integration into the Russian Federation's sociocultural space. Specialists in the field of psychological counseling can be found everywhere: preschool and educational institutions and firms, various social and psychological centers and other institutions and organizations.

At present, psychological counselors work in the fields of individual, family, age-specific, organizational and other types of counseling. In Russia, the non-profit organization "Federation of Psychological

Counselors of Russia" has been created with the aim of setting up local psychological counseling units.

The need for this kind of assistance is beyond question. Practically from the first meeting, it helps clients to get answers to their questions and find their own solutions to problems using the resources available at the moment.

REFERENCES

Abramova, G. S. (2000). *Vvedenie v prakticheskuyu psihologiyu* [*Introduction to Practical Psychology*] G. S. Abramova. – Ekaterinburg : Delovaya Kniga Publ. 237 pp.

Abramova, G. S. (2005). *Praktikum po psihologicheskomu konsul'tirovaniyu* [*Tutorial on Psychological Counseling*] G. S. Abramova. – Ekaterinburg : Delovaya Kniga Publ. 119 pp.

Aleshina, Y. E. (2003). Individual'noe i semejnoe psihologicheskoe konsul'tirovanie [Individual and Family Psychological Counseling] Y. E. Aleshina. – Moscow : RID "*Soc. zdorov'e Rossii*". 176 pp.

Bubnova, S. S. (2000). Psihologicheskie aspekty professional'noj konsul'tacii [Psychological Aspects of Professional Counseling] *Psihologicheskij zhurnal*. 144 pp.

Burmenskaya, G. V., Karabanova, O. A. & Lidere, A. G. (2002). *Vozrastno-psihologicheskoe konsul'tirovanie* [*Age-specific Psychological Counseling*]/G. V. Burmenskaya, O. A. Karabanova, A. G. Lidere. Moscow: Akademiya Publ. 416 pp.

Cerbin, V. P. & Lepezhenkova, L. N. (2004). *Opyt psihologicheskoj konsul'tacii v Hartmann, E*. 1997. The Concept of Boundaries in Counselling and Ppsychotherapy. *British Journal of Guidance & Counselling*, *25*(2), P. 147-162.

Heppner, P., Leong, F. T. L. & Chiao, H. A. (2008). Growing Internationalization of Counseling Psychology. In: Brown, S. D. & Lent, R. W. *Handbook of Counseling Psychology* (4th ed). New York: Wiley.

Klyueva, N. V. (2011). *Konsul'tacionnaya psihologiya: metodicheskie ukazaniya* [*Psychological Counseling: Guidelines*] N. V. Klyueva; Yarosl. gos. un-t im. P. G. Demidova. Yaroslavl': Yaroslavl' State University. 60 pp.

Nikolova, N., Möllering, G. & Reihlen, M. (2015). Trusting as a "Leap of Faith": Trust-building Practices in Client–Consultant Relationships. *Scandinavian Journal of Management*, *31*(2), 232-245.

Psihologiya. Uchebnik dlya gumanitarnyh vuzov [*Psychology. Textbook for Liberal Arts Higher Educational Institutions*] 2001. Pod obshchej red. V. N. Druzhinina. St. Petersburg: Piter Publ. 656 pp.

Rogers, C. R. (1957). The necessary and sufficient conditions of therapeutic personality change. *Journal of Consulting Psychology*, *21*, 95–103.

Ronch, Judah L., William van Ornum, & Nicholas C. Stilwell, eds. (1994). *The Counseling Sourcebook: A Practical Reference on Contemporary Issues*. New York : Crossroad.

Vernon, Ann, ed. (1993). *Counseling Children and Adolescents*. Denver, CO: Love.

Woolfe, Ray, et al. (2003). Counselling Psychology in Context. *Handbook of Counselling Psychology*, 2nd ed., Sage Publications.

In: Psychological Service …
Editor: Svitlana V. Kucherenko
ISBN: 978-1-53618-160-9

Chapter 10

DIRECTIONS OF THE UNIVERSITY PSYCHOLOGICAL SERVICE' WORK: EDUCATIONAL ACTIVITIES IN THE SYSTEM OF PSYCHOLOGICAL SUPPORT OF HIGHER EDUCATION

Georgiy P. Grigoriev*[*]*, MD
Psychology Department,
V.I. Vernadsky Crimean Federal University, Crimea, Russia

ABSTRACT

The Chapter is devoted to the problem of psychological education in the system of psychological support of students of higher educational institutions. The theoretical construct "psychological culture" is analyzed. Psychological culture is a part of the General culture of a person, which involves the development of a system of knowledge in the field of basic scientific psychology, basic skills in understanding the characteristics of

[*] Corresponding Author's Email: geogrig@rambler.ru.

the psyche (your own and others), and the use of this knowledge in everyday life. It is concluded that psychological education of teachers and students is an important component of psychological support of the pedagogical process in higher education.

Keywords: psychological support, psychological culture, psychological education, psychological prophylaxis, personality-oriented approach

INTRODUCTION

Over the past decade the educational system of the Russian Federation has undergone significant changes, which have led to a change in the paradigm of its construction – developing education has entered the real practice of education, which has ceased to be only a scientific concept. "Developmental education is not only a varied, heterogeneous or unified education, but primarily education focused on the development of individual capabilities, abilities and interests of students, that is, personality-oriented education. It cannot be built on the paradigm of a simple transfer of knowledge and skills, but it presupposes a special organization of a developing educational space based on personality-oriented pedagogical technologies"(Rubtsov V.V. 2006)

Personally oriented education for its implementation requires, firstly, significant individualization of education in the form of developing new educational content, creating new basic curricula, adopting modern educational standards that ensure matching education with real needs of different groups of students, taking into account their cultural, national and economic life. Secondly, the development of new methods and forms of academic work, including training and education, the widespread use of modern computer technologies and Internet technologies is necessary.

According to Rubtsov V.V., academician of the Russian Academy of Education, director of the Psychological Institute of the Russian Academy of Education, the rationale for constructing a basic psychological education program can be based on the following:

"Firstly, the program of such training should be reasonably balanced between a package of general fundamental courses and its practice-oriented (significant in volume) part.

Secondly, in the context of the well-known uncertainty and complexity of the graduate's future work, preference should be given to the universal training of a psychologist who can work both independently and in a certain professional capacity (for example, as a psycho-diagnosis, consultant, psychologist of distant learning), and be included in the work the whole team.

Thirdly, the latter circumstance determines the balance of academic hours between the general training program for students and disciplines of narrow specialization in favor of the former.

Fourth, the functions of such a psychologist suggest the prevalence of the development of specific technologies of professional activity over research and theoretical work. A graduate of the Faculty of Psychology must be able to do and act, i.e., in a good way, be an applied project-oriented psychologist.

Fifth, the psychologist should receive serious training in the field of pedagogical psychology (including psychological theories of learning, the psychological foundations of modern educational systems, new educational, including computer technologies), which will allow him to solve the problems of interacting with teachers in the process educational activities, building and supporting educational environments, examination and analysis of concepts, technologies, decisions made with a view to their compliance with the development tasks of specific contingents of children. Moreover, the knowledge gained during the preparation process must be mastered by him in the form of specific techniques, technologies and methods of action, as well as the possibility of their application in a new situation "(Rubtsov V.V., 2006, 2008).

The most important aspect in the educational process of higher education is psychological and pedagogical support. Based on a theoretical study and semantic analysis of conceptual interpretations, Raskalinos, V. (2016) offers his own definition of the psychological and pedagogical support of the educational process, emphasizes the importance of supporting the personal development of students and their effective overcoming difficulties encountered in the learning process, and focuses on the interests of students and maintaining the integrity of their inner world. The author comes to the conclusion that it is necessary to develop the content of psychological and pedagogical support of the educational process, taking into account the existing requirements of the federal state educational standard and the expectations of society.

Interesting results were obtained by Terada, T. & Kasai, M. & Asano, K. (2006) when substantiating the need for psychological support for high school students. It turned out that the older children in the family received psychological support from mother and father to a greater extent than the younger ones. In addition, older boys received significantly greater psychological support from both parents than younger boys or girls. The revealed differences require an individual approach with psychological and pedagogical support of students.

Moreover, according to O.A. Rudakova (2016), "a personality-oriented approach is considered as fundamental in the organization of psychological support for the development of the personality of student youth, which needs special attention and the help of a psychologist during the training at a higher educational institution, has a wide range of personality and interpersonal problems arising from social and economic transformations of modern society."

In technological terms, psychological support acts as a system of tools that contain various forms, methods and techniques of psychological assistance to the development of students' personalities, including psychological education.

METHODS

General Concepts of Psychological Education

The concept of "psychological education" is interpreted in different ways in literary and reference sources. One of the earliest definitions is proposed by K.K. Platonov: "Psychological problems of propaganda are determined by the capabilities of psychological science to help to increase the effectiveness of propaganda as the main form of ideological work by taking into account the psychological regularities of the influence of the propagandist's personality and his advocacy, in particular taking into account the psychological characteristics of speech communication" (Platonov K.K. 1984). However, this definition relates more to the features of propaganda activities than to psychological education. V. V. Pakhalian gives a general definition of education: "education is directed to the timely and targeted distribution of information to prevent the appearance of typical difficulties in development, in mastering activities, in the communication of children, etc." (Pakhalian V. V. 2002, p. 41).

A brief definition of "psychological education" was first given by I. V. Dubrovina: "Psychological education is the familiarization of adults (educators, teachers, parents) and children with psychological knowledge" (Dubrovina I. V. 1991, p. 59). The author sees the main point of this work in:

1) "familiarization of educators, teachers and parents with the basic laws and conditions for the favorable development of the child;
2) popularization and clarification of the results of the latest psychological research;
3) the formation of the need for psychological knowledge, the desire to use them in working with a child or in the interests of developing one's own personality;
4) familiarization of students with the basics of self-knowledge, self-education;
5) achieving an understanding of the need for practical psychology and the work of a psychologist in a children's educational institution" (Dubrovina I. V.: 1991, p. 59).

Thus, the main way and at the same time one of the active forms of realizing the tasks of psycho prophylactic work in the activity of a practical psychologist is psychological education, regardless of which system he works in (education, healthcare, industry, law enforcement, etc.

The content of psychological education is determined based on the specifics, type and profile of the institution. It can be considered as a direction of practice-oriented psychology, and its purpose is the transfer and dissemination of psychological knowledge. Psychological education can be considered as the primary form of people's involvement in psychological knowledge.

In general, we can conclude that psychological education (Chuprov L.F. 2013) is a type of preventive activity of a specialist psychologist aimed at forming positive attitudes toward psychological assistance, the activities of a practical psychologist among general public (teachers, educators, schoolchildren, parents), broadening the horizons in the field of psychological knowledge.

Based on this definition, we can conclude that psychological education performs three tasks:

- the first task is the formation of scientific attitudes and ideas about psychological science and practical psychology (psychologization of society);
- the second task is to inform the population on issues of psychological knowledge;
- third one is the formation of a sustainable need for the application and use of psychological knowledge in order to effectively socialize the younger generation and for their own development (Chuprov. L.F. 2013).

According to L.F. Chuprov, options for psychological enlightenment in education can be active when the active subject of education (propaganda of psychological enlightenment, campaigning for the introduction and use of scientific psychological knowledge and clarification of the need for psychological assistance, etc.) is the psychologist himself, and not a formal one, which involves only informing upon customer request.

As I.A. Egorova (2010) rightly observes, "the process of any activity is triggered by the corresponding motivation, therefore the basis of psychological education is the formation of the desire to acquire psychological knowledge and the desire to use it in life and practical activities. This aspiration, in turn, has a cognitive basis - a system of ideas about psychology as a science and sphere of practical activity.

The need for psychological education is also due to the fact that among the population, including students studying not in psychological specialties, psychology is associated with a number of myths and misconceptions.

I.A. Egorova cites some of the myths that one has to face in the process of enlightenment: "The main phrase of a psychologist is "Do you want to talk about this?"; "The psychologist will solve all your problems without your participation;" "The psychologist is a man without problems;" "The psychologist is always in a good mood"; "Psychologists are extraordinary personalities (either a genius-sage, or with an abnormal psyche)"; "The psychologist gives advice on what to do"; "It is enough for a psychologist to look at a person to find out everything about him"; "Sigmund Freud came up with the whole psychology."

Psychological education aims to replace various myths with scientific knowledge.

FORMS OF PSYCHOLOGICAL EDUCATION

Various forms are used, such as mass actions or direct contacts in psychological education. The effectiveness of mass psychological education is difficult to evaluate. In direct contact in the process of psychological counseling it is much easier to evaluate its effectiveness or inefficiency, since in this case it is possible to highlight the effect of psychological impact.

Many authors attribute the following to the main forms of psychological education:

- verbal (conversation, lecture, speech on the radio, on television),
- journalism (print and electronic media),
- visual (poster, booklet, memo),

- interactive, etc.
- use the Internet for psychological education (placement of thematic information on web-sites, etc.).

Let us consider in detail some of the forms of psychological education.

Conversation. According to K.K. Platonov, "Conversation is one of the basic general methods of psychological science, providing for direct or indirect oral receipt information from the studied person by verbal communication with him about his activities, in which the inherent mental phenomena are objectified " (Platonov K.K. 1984, p. 16).

"The forms of conversation are also different:

- the lecturer tells and occasionally addresses the audience (inactive form);
- the lecturer announces the problem around which the discussion will take place, listeners express their opinions, it is important not only to give an assessment (right or wrong, good or bad), the main thing is to substantiate their arguments, only the right justification can lead to the right conclusions made independently;
- in the process of work, an artificially created situation allows categorical objections or approval, which causes an active and prompt reaction from the audience;
- by agreement with the students, with the aim of everyone participating in the discussion of this problem, one part of the students asks questions, another one answers, and vice versa;
- one part of the students names specific situations, the other part justifies how much the given examples of situations correspond to a problem or a question" (Chuprov L.F. 2013).

As we emphasized above, the most effective form of psychological enlightenment in education is an individual conversation. In this regard, each communication of a psychologist with a person, when a psychologist exercises his professional duties, performs the function of education. This version of education is usually not planned in advance and is largely informal. The content of the conversation is determined by the specific request of the client and the preliminary conclusions obtained from the psychological examination. Compliance with ethical standards and pedagogical tact is the main requirement for conversation in any of its specific cases.

Lecture. As L.F. Chuprov points out, "The lecture presupposes a consistent presentation of educational (methodological, scientific) material. The main didactic requirements for the lecture are as follows:

- high scientific and theoretical level (taking into account the preparedness of the audience);
- holistic disclosure of the topic;
- analysis of specific facts and phenomena in their relationship; their generalization;
- connection with previously studied material: emotional presentation, etc. "(Chuprov L.F. 2013).

It is well known that the psychologist in his practical activities everywhere carries out the communicative process, i.e., is a communication specialist. However, if during psychological communication the psychologist shows only the desire to communicate and expressiveness, not supplemented by thought and competence, such work will not bring much benefit. Excellent knowledge of the material, general erudition, the ability to convey even the most complex material to an untrained listener comes first. This greatly contributes to the effectiveness of psychological education. Is it necessary for a psychologist to master oratory? L.F. Chuprov answers this question this way: "Actually a great oratory in psychological education is not required. If there is no gift that ignites the audience, orator- lecturer, you can replace this with the reception of a lecturer – interlocutor, involving in communication and updating the experience of specific members of the audience. The manner of presentation of the material and the very attitude of the communicator to the audience also play an important role. To date, a large arsenal of concrete forms of its holding has been accumulated in psychological education" (Chuprov L.F. 2013).

Publication of articles on psychological issues. The publication of articles on psychological issues in various contemporary magazines on current topics, such as how to deal with stress, how to gain confidence in communicating with others, how to stay calm if something hurts you a lot can be another form of psychological education. The peculiarity of publication, even in a magazine which is popular among young people, has the peculiarity that the information in the article remains unidirectional without the necessary feedback. In this regard, publications on the sites of social groups differ for the better, where the publication of a psychologist on a relevant topic can cause a stream of comments and "likes."

Some television programs, in which psychologists discuss important issues, are also popular. However, in this case, caution and sobriety must be exercised, since among these programs there are also absolutely unscientific, filled with mystery and mysticism.

Visual forms of psychological education are posters, special showcases, psychological leaflets and booklets. These forms migrated to the office of the psychologist from preventive medical propaganda. You remember posters "Wash hands before eating," "When a flu epidemic, wear a gauze bandage," etc. You can imagine a poster calling to be mutually polite (such ones sometimes occur). Obviously, firstly they have an "interior" function, and they play a role in psychological education only in the second (third) place.

At the same time, certain topical issues that excite students, and most clearly worked out by a psychologist can be arranged in the form of small brochures multiplied on a printer. They can be handed out in training groups. In general, we can conclude that most of these visuals have low informational usefulness, but they can always be presented to inspectors.

Thus, it is obvious that direct communication and predominantly oral verbal forms of information and education are more effective in practical psychology.

Keep in mind that the essence of psychological education as a whole lies in the formation and development of the psychological culture of the individual. It is necessary to dwell on this statement in detail.

L.S. Kolmogorova (2001) proposed the definition of psychological culture as "an integral part of a person's basic culture, which is a complex-structured formation that allows him to understand the person's inner world, effectively solve psychological problems of life, adapt and self-determine in a society that promotes self-realization, self-development, harmonization of the inner world and relations with others, generating a state of inner well-being"(Kolmogorova LS. 2001, pp. 11-12).

"Psychological culture is an important component of the general harmony of the personality, such a broad aspect of it as the general culture of vital activity and the functioning of the personality" (Motkov O.I. 1999).

O.I. Motkov defines psychological culture as "a personality characteristic that expresses in a developed form a rather high quality of self-organization and self-regulation of any human activity, various types of its basic aspirations and tendencies, personality relationships (towards oneself, close and distant people, live and inanimate nature, the world in general) "(Motkov O.I. 1999).

"The psychological culture of the personality includes a complex of many components:

- developed special aspirations, orientations, originally inherent in a man in the form of special motivational tendencies;
- natural abilities that ensure the implementation of cultural and psychological aspirations;
- intravital skills and steadily and daily manifesting types of behavior corresponding to these aspirations and abilities "(Klimov E.A. 2000).

Allakhverdov V.M. et al., (1985) emphasize "an understanding of practical problems that psychologists can solve; understanding of the specifics of psychological analysis of behavior (as opposed to the analysis of everyday life); constant striving for self-knowledge and self-improvement as components of the psychological culture of a professional."

Klimov E.A. (2000) claims that "psychological culture is a part of the general culture of a person (as a family member, citizen, specialist), which involves the development of a knowledge system in the field of the basics of scientific psychology, basic skills in understanding the characteristics of the psyche (one's own and those around him) the use of this knowledge in everyday life, in self-education and professional activity."

From the point of view of Obozov N.N. three components must be included in the concept of psychological culture: "understanding and knowledge of oneself and other people; adequate self-esteem and assessment of other people; self-regulation of personal states and properties, self-regulation of activity, regulation of relations with other people"(Obozov N.N. 1986).

According to Egorova. I.A., "the role of psychological education in the system of professional activity of a psychologist lies, first of all, in creating a motivational basis for the formation and development of the psychological culture of the individual. The main goals of the educational work of a psychologist are to create adequate ideas about psychology as a science and field of practical activity, about the possibilities of a practical psychologist, which will ultimately lead to the awareness of the population of the need for psychological knowledge and skills and the expansion of the psychological services market"(Egorova I.A. 2010).

Enlightenment of teachers. Psychological education of teachers is another important component of the psychological support of studying at a university. Psychological education in this direction is aimed at such work in which every teacher could gain the knowledge of psychology that he needs in his professional activities. These knowledge and skills will allow teachers to organize an effective process of teaching their subject from both a substantive and a methodological point of view; psychologically competently build relationships with students and colleagues on psychologically competent foundations.

The basic principle of educating teachers can be formulated as follows: a combination of practical activities for transferring knowledge to students and the process of obtaining psychological knowledge by the teacher. That is, psychological and educational work should be coupled with the current extracurricular activities of the departments (scientific and methodological seminars on psychological topics).

PSYCHOLOGICAL EDUCATION AND PSYCHOLOGICAL PROPHYLAXIS

Psychological education can be considered as one of the forms of solving psycho prophylactic tasks. As shown above, an important place in the system of psychological support of the educational process is held by psychological education. However, if we talk about psycho prophylaxis, then its tasks can be successfully solved only with the interaction of specialists and social institutions. On the contrary, psychological education is a direct duty, and a relatively independent active form of activity in the psycho prophylactic work of a practical psychologist working in an educational institution.

Obviously, many social factors contribute to the personal development of a person, having a positive effect on him. At the same time, there are also such factors that have a negative effect on the individual and lead to disharmony of behavior, including the "anomaly" of the person (meaning substance abuse, drug addiction, etc.) in the society. Similar situations in the life of a young man require painstaking psycho prophylactic work aimed at forming the individual's resistance to the destructive influences of the social environment. Psychological education and psychological awareness help the young man to navigate the complex diversity of life around him.

It is also necessary to take into account in psychoprophylactic work, that difficulties of a social, economic and domestic nature lead to the fact that a young person has a higher level of neuroticism, anxiety, and an increased interest in mysticism. Hence it is natural that young people begin to seek help from various psychics and sorcerers. It was revealed that almost 80% of young people, who fall into the networks of banned religious organizations, relying in their activities on ignorance, lack of information, inexperience of young people.

In solving these problems, the tasks that are performed by social educators and practical educational psychologists intersect.

Officially, the main activities of the teacher-psychologist are psycho diagnostics, psycho-correctional work, psychological counseling and organizational and methodological work. One of the important areas of work of a psychologist is psycho prophylaxis. However, in reality, in textbooks and manuals intended for training a practical psychologist, it is not actually described.

Must be emphasized that psychological education is necessary for all members of society, but first of all it should be aimed at those who, due to a lack of education, specific work or everyday life, were unprepared to master and actively use psychological knowledge in their life activities (Alferov A.D. et al., 1984).

The presented review of literary sources on the problem of psychological education in the system of psychological support for students in institutions of higher education allows us to draw some conclusions.

Firstly, psychological education is a necessary component of psychological support for students.

Secondly, in psychological education at a university it is advisable to use time-tested forms and methods of psychological education: conversations, lectures, publications in mass media and on the Internet.

Thirdly, psychological education should be aimed at creating a common culture of students.

Fourth, psychological education should be coupled with psycho prophylactic activity at the university.

And finally, psychological education can only be effectively carried out by being integrated into the overall system of the educational process at a university.

References

Alferov A.D. et al., 1984. *Osnovy metodicheskogo obespecheniya pedagogicheskogo vseobucha roditeley (metodicheskiye rekomendatsii)* [*Fundamentals of methodological support for pedagogical universal education of parents (guidelines).*] Sostav.: A.D. Alferov, V.V. Bogza, V.G. Pavlenko, V.G. Fotov. Rostov-na-Donu. 69 pp.

Allakhverdov V.M. et al., 1985. *O formirovanii psikhologicheskoy kultury u studentov tekhnicheskogo vuza* [*On the formation of psychological culture among students of a technical university*]. V.M. Allakhverdov. N.V. Belyak. M.V. Ivanov. Psikhologicheskoye obespecheniye uchebno-vospitatelnogo protsessa v vuze: Mezhvuzovskiy sbornik. L.

Chuprov L.F.. 2013. Psikhologicheskoye prosveshcheniye v sisteme psikhoprofilakticheskoy raboty prakticheskogo psikhologa: Osnovy teorii i metodika [Psychological education in the system of psychoprophylactic work of a practical psychologist: Fundamentals of theory and methodology]. PEM: *Psychology. Educology. Medicine*. № 1.sr; 75 pp. URL: pem.esrae.ru/1-7. (data obrashcheniya: 18.12.2019).

Dubrovina I.V. 1991. Psikhologicheskoye prosveshcheniye [Psychological education]. Shkolnaya psikhologicheskaya sluzhba: voprosy teorii i praktiki. – *M. Pedagogika*. 1991. Pp.138–139.

Egorova I.A. 2010. Psikhologicheskoye prosveshcheniye v sisteme professionalnoy deyatelnosti psikhologa [Psychological education in the system of professional activity of a psychologist]. *Vestnik TIUiE*. 2010. №1. URL: https://cyberleninka.ru/article/n/psihologicheskoe-prosveschenie-v-sisteme-professionalnoy-deyatelnosti-psihologa (data obrashcheniya: 18.12.2019).

Klimov. E.A. 2000. *Psikhologiya: vospitaniye. Obucheniye* [*Psychology: education, training*]. E. A. Klimov. M. YuNITI-DANA.

Kolmogorova. L.S. 2001. *Vozrastnyye vozmozhnosti i osobennosti stanovleniya psikhologicheskoy kultury uchashchikhsya* [*Age-related opportunities and features of the formation of psychological culture of students*]: Avtoref. dis. ... d-ra psikh nauk. M.

Motkov O.I. 1999. Psikhologicheskaya kultura lichnosti [Psychological personality culture]. *Shkolnyy psikholog*. №15. Pp. 8 – 9.

Obozov N.N. 1986. *Psikhologicheskaya kultura vzaimnykh otnosheniy* [*The psychological culture of mutual relations.*] N.N. Obozov – L.

Pakhalian V.V. 2002. Psikhoprofilaktika v obrazovanii [Psychological prophylaxis in education]. V.V. Pakhalian. *Voprosy psikhologii*. № 1. P. 38–44.

Platonov K.K. 1984. Kratkiy slovar sistemy psikhologicheskikh ponyatiy [Brief dictionary of the system of psychological concepts]. M. "*Vysshaya shkola*." 174 pp.

Raskalinos V. 2016. Vektor nauki Tol'yattinskogo gosudarstvennogo universiteta [Psychological and pedagogical support of the educational process]. *Seriya Pedagogika i psihologiya*. 11-15. 10.18323/2221-5662-2016-4-11-15.

Rubtsov. V.V. 2006. *Psikhologicheskoye obespecheniye novoy paradigmy obrazovaniya i novykh obrazovatelnykh tekhnologiy* (elektronnyy resurs) [*Psychological support of the new paradigm of education and new educational technologies* (electronic resource)]. URL: https:// works.doklad.ru/view/ G41FGYSqMRk.html (data obrashcheniya: 18.12.2019).

Rubtsov V.V. 2008. Sovremennoe psikhologicheskoe obrazovanie: problemy i perspektivy. *Sbornik materialov konferentsii "Psikholog i obshchestvo: dialog o vzaimodeistvii*" [Modern psychological education: problems and prospects. *Proceedings of conference* "*Psychologist and society: A Dialogue on cooperation*"]. (Moscow, 12 fevralya 2008) Moscow, 47 pp.

Rudakova. O.A. 2016. Psikhologicheskoye soprovozhdeniye v vysshikh obrazovatelnykh uchrezhdeniyakh [Psychological support in higher educational institutions]. O.A. Rudakova Nauchno-pedagogicheskoye obozreniye. *Pedagogical Review*. – 4 (14). – S. 18–26.

Terada, Tomonori & Kasai, Makiko & Asano, Koji. 2006. Psychological support for junior high school students: Sibling order and sex. *Psychological reports*. 99. 179-190.

In: Psychological Service …
Editor: Svitlana V. Kucherenko
ISBN: 978-1-53618-160-9

Chapter 11

DIRECTIONS OF THE UNIVERSITY PSYCHOLOGICAL SERVICE' WORK: POSSIBILITIES OF UNIVERSITY STUDENTS' DEEP PSYCHOLOGICAL CORRECTION

Oksana N. Usatenko*, PhD and Maria S. Maik†, PhD
V. I. Vernadsky Crimean Federal University,
Simferopol, Crimea, Russia/Ukraine

ABSTRACT

The article highlights the theoretical and methodological justification and results of deep psychological correction with University students according to the author's method of T. Yatsenko. The article reveals the peculiarities of interpretation the phenomenon of psychological correction in its individual and group versions. The article deepens the understanding of group dynamics and its specifics in the process of deep psychological correction.

* Corresponding Author's Email: usatekoxana@mail.ru.
† Corresponding Author's Email: live.psiholog@mail.ru.

Keywords: deep psychological correction, methodology, active social and psychological principles (ASPP), personal problem, effectiveness of deep psychological correction

INTRODUCTION

The Russian Federation has historically been a multi-ethnic region, which suggests the importance of creating a multicultural educational space for modern learning youth. One of the most important tasks of higher education is the problem of both socio-cultural and psychological acculturation, which is characterized by a set of internal psychological consequences (a clear sense of personal or cultural identity, good psychological health and achievement of psychological satisfaction in a new cultural context).

It is established that the factors affecting psychological and socio-cultural acculturation are interrelated. They include personal characteristics, life events, social support, cultural knowledge, the level of involvement in contacts and intergroup aspirations.

The development of adaptive capabilities of students is especially important for their educational and professional integration into the social space of the University against the background of psychological characteristics of the youth age period.

The purpose of our work is to present the work results on the development of the adaptive potential of students of the Academy of humanities and pedagogy by means of deep psychological correction.

Psychological correction is generally understood as a set of psychological means used by a psychologist to correct the shortcomings of mentally healthy person psychology or behavior. Specific features of the psychological correction process are: the orientation to a clinically healthy personality of people who have psychological difficulties, problems, complaints of a neurotic nature in their daily life, as well as people who feel good, but want to change their lives or set a goal for personal development; the orientation of psychological corrective impacts on behavior change and development of the client's personality; the orientation to the healthy sides of the personality regardless of the degree of impairment. Psychological correction deals with already formed personality qualities or behaviors and is aimed at changing them.

Psychological correction is used in two forms: individual and group. The advantages of individual psychological correction include confidentiality, which contributes to removing psychological barriers and self-disclosure of the client. It is believed that this type of psychological correction is ineffective in solving interpersonal problems that require working in a group. The specificity of psychological correction group is in targeted use of group dynamics, i.e., the entire set of relationships and interactions occurring between the group members and the psychologist for correctional purposes.

A psychological correction group is an artificially created small group united by the goals of interpersonal research, personal learning, and self-disclosure in a "here and now" situation. In this situation participants study the processes of interpersonal interaction at a given moment and in a given place. Group psychological correction considers the client in a socio-psychological context, in the context of his relationships and interactions with others. This helps to push the boundaries of the correction process and focus not only on the individual and his intrapersonal problems, but on the individual real relationships and interactions with the world around him. The relationships and interactions that the client enters into in the group largely reflect his true relationships. The group acts as a model of real life, where the client shows the same attitudes, aspirations, values, the same ways of emotional and behavioral response.

The use of group dynamics is aimed at ensuring that each participant has the opportunity to express himself, and creating an effective feedback system that allows the client to understand himself more adequately and deeply, to see his own inadequate relationships and aspirations, emotional behavioral patterns, manifested in interpersonal interaction, and change them in an atmosphere of goodwill and mutual acceptance. Group dynamics is provided by specific organizational principles of the group.

Methods

Group Variant of Deep-Correction Work

The article presents the results of a group variant of deep-correction work in the author's version of T. Yatsenko's psychodynamic approach (Yacenko, T., Polianychko, O. and Pedchenko, O. (2016), Galushko L., Dmeterko N., Yevtushenko I., Maksimenko E., Pedchenko A., Polyanichko E., Tuz L., Usatenko O. (2012). The psychodynamic approach as a whole is characterized by solving issues related to the dynamic aspects of the psyche, i.e., motives, drives, urges, internal conflicts (contradictions), the existence and development of which ensure the functioning and development of the personal "Self." The central concept for representatives of the psychodynamic approach in understanding the causes of behavior disorders and the client's emotional life is a "conflict." Thus, the main task of the psychodynamic approach is bringing to the client's consciousness a conflict situation related to the inadmissibility of unconscious cravings for him. It is assumed that awareness of the presence of unconscious impulses and the conflict situation itself is the way to solve these conflicts.

The effectiveness of psychological correction group involves a deep understanding of the features of mental destructions, and their connection with the subject's Edipal dependencies. These dependencies are masked by protection and are not realized, preserving the energy potential for influencing behavior. From a practical point of view, the subject of analysis is such individual behavior, which carries the potential for conflict, regression and generates not only internal discomfort, but also tension, difficulties in relationships with other people. The group creates conditions for studying the features of the internal, implicitly hidden from consciousness determination of the subject's behavior imperatively affecting behavior in any communication situation (household or office).

The study of internal conditioning of behavior is facilitated by a group atmosphere contributing to spontaneity and involuntary behavior, while minimizing instructional urges to action. This opens up prospects of learning uncontrollable internal aspirations that actively affect the nature and content of communication. So, the object of attention of a professional psychologist in a psychological correction group is the facts of discrepancy between deliberately declared goals, motives, aspirations for action and the very nature of the subject's action (behavior). It is also important to distinguish between behavior contrary to the declared purpose, the deep content of which is hidden from the subject, because of demonstrative behavior.

The prerequisites for group dynamics include the mandatory introduction by the head of group and acceptance by the participants of group principles of work aimed at creating a specific atmosphere conducive to self-disclosure and self-knowledge of the group members. The following principles apply in a deep-oriented psychological correction group.

1) The principle of voluntariness is that the client makes his own decision to work in the corrective group, because he is personally interested in his own changes. In the conditions of the university, this principle is implemented with certain restrictions, because the student is required to attend a group. Therefore, at the beginning of the group's work, the head suggests to voice their own goals that can be achieved in the course of work, adjusting them for realism and. Thus, it helps to actualize the internal motivation of a person, since it is impossible to make somebody change if he does not want to, but it is possible to arouse interest in his own development.

   According to the principles of group work, everyone can refuse any exercise if he feels difficulties in performing it, but the head of the group encourages participants to overcome internal barriers. At the same time, it should be understood that barriers are a sign of resistances that need to be overcome.
2) The principle of confidentiality is in keeping a group personal information inside the group. Participants can analyze or present group information both within the group and outside it, in terms of

the effectiveness of forms and methods of work, since the group also performs a didactic function. However, group members should not discuss outside the group or in between what is going on in the group because they deprive the group of important information material.

3) The principle of unbiased judgement implies no criticism or appraisal opinions in black and white categories. It deals with total acceptance of the person and doesn't involve unnecessary wishes, advices, categories of "good" or "bad," comparison with each other. At first, mutual acceptance of each other can be difficult, especially for separate members of the group. Such difficulties are forestalled by an atmosphere of trust in the group. The more spontaneous, involuntary statements there are, the more optimal the group atmosphere is for learning. In each situation, it is advisable for the group members to be emotionally liberated and open, to get rid of the tension and fear of punishment that can restrain activity in the "here and now" situation.
4) The principle of equality includes referring to "you" and by name, both between participants and the head of the group. Participants also has the ability to "engage" in the group process as a group leader, if necessary. That is, the psychological correction group is nondirective.
5) The "here and now" principle. It is desirable to "draw" situations from a past life not only verbally, but also to model its plot with the help of role-playing participation of group members. Actions, deeds, and activity in the "here and now" situation have the greatest value in analyzing the material. Group work is associated with certain emotional loads which are involuntarily actualized under the influence of "traces" of past experience. Group members learn about the features of the group process as an integral system of psychological and pedagogical impact on the individual, which is formed spontaneously, involuntarily, with a touch of emotional exertion.

6) The principle of spontaneity and involuntary behavior. Relaxed behavior, sincerity and sensitivity in relationships are appreciated in the group. The deep-correction group has an unconventional character, both in terms of indirect forms of group management, and rules of behavior of group members, which are characterized by the absence of strict regulation of behavior and the acceptability of spontaneous and involuntary forms of it.
7) The feedback principle suggests talking about your feelings, rather than evaluating them, as well as evaluating your actions. Thanks to feedback (on an emotional and sensory level), each member of the group can evaluate his strengths and potential. Qualities that are undesirable should not be pushed out of consciousness, it is better to make efforts to accept them and learn them in the process of self-improvement.
8) The principle of confrontation. Criticism as a working tool is not used psychological correction in group. Close to criticism is the feedback in the form of confrontation. Going into a confrontation with another member of the group means telling him openly and sincerely about something important in terms of personal self-discovery but not very pleasant for him. Thus, the group members significantly help each other in finding important conclusions and solutions. A sincere, immediate reaction may not be very pleasant to the other person. At the same time, it is important not to offend each other and to find optimal forms of presenting information without impoverishing its content. This practice is also an element of coaching the acceptability of behaviors in communication. If you learn to find the optimal form of sincere expression of your thoughts and feelings, even if they are not very pleasant to the interlocutor – this is the way to learn and train your communication skills.
9) The principle of activity. A group member has the right to refuse a particular exercise in the group, although self-blocking of activity is not desirable, it is proposed to remove (level) person's own blocks.

10) The principle of frankness and sincerity. The key to successful training in group psychological correction is an atmosphere of frankness, but not in the usual sense of it, when the innermost secrets are revealed, but as a frank expression of one's own reaction to the situation "here and now." If one of the group members has a desire to share intimate aspects of his problems in hope to understand them better, then this can be accepted in the context of group integration. Self-disclosure, according to the ASPP (active social and psychological principles), is not mandatory. More important is the sincerity of reactions to what is happening in the group in the "here and now" situation.

The implementation of these principles by itself is difficult for many clients. These difficulties can be a topic for discussion in the group and the subject of psychological correction study. Elaboration and acceptance of these principles is important in the context of mastering the ethical standards of the psychologist's work at the stage of professionalization.

Thanks to the development of acceptable forms of behavior among the participants, the group gradually integrates, becomes a single whole, and each of its members brings something unique with their own freedom of behavior. The group process may develop unevenly in terms of its intensity. This should not be a cause for concern, the artificial stimulation of activity is not desirable. The group process has its own internal dynamics.

The process of deep psychological correction is not strictly regulated, and the standard management style is not acceptable here, although the group members traditionally may have such expectations. Optimal cognitive material is provided with relaxed, spontaneous behavior. It is undesirable to analyze events and situations that go beyond the scope of group work (movies, household stories, etc.). This is seen as a kind of "leaving the group." It is important for everyone in a group to learn to trust themselves, their own spontaneity, and to master the skills of free behavior.

Group relationships that develop in the substantive work conditions with no prosocial goals actualize irrational behavior caused by "protective" tendencies of the Self. At the same time, any manifestations of the subject's psyche – utterance, nonverbal behavior, psycho-drawing – carry the possibility of actualization of involuntary emotional reactions, which contributes to mutual knowledge. Relationships that arise in the group reveal the stereotypical behavior, which is involved in the formation of psychological defenses. It is the spontaneously actualized relationship model that provides opportunities to study the personality deformations of each member of the group, which are hidden from consciousness and self-control.

The personal problem of the individual objectively contains the presence of an internal contradiction, which is objectified in the divergence of the logic of the conscious and the logic of the unconscious (Usatenko O. 2014). At the same time, there is a departure from reality, as well as distortions of social-perceptual reality and replacing objective reality with a psychic one. The last is loaded with certain illusory representations in unison with the system of psychological protection. The consistency of psychological defenses is their essential characteristic, which is manifested on the spontaneous behavioral material. This is due to the fact that these characteristics objectify the logic of the unconscious, which has the opposite direction to the logic of consciousness, declared by the individual. The logic of the unconscious, or "other logic," is an indicator of the functioning of the basal form of psychological protection. Being in close relationship with situational (peripheral) defenses, they have a certain autonomy and are more dependent on the unconscious aspects of the psyche than on the tasks of prosocial self-realization.

The personal problem is not recognized by the subject, so it is difficult to achieve its solution. The psychologist helps the individual discover it and transfer it from the implicit level to the explicit one. The subject is only aware of the consequences of having a personal problem (anxiety, tension, increased aggressiveness, etc.). Knowledge of the deep origins of personal difficulties and problems is associated with psychological protection, which sets a specific, individually unique dynamics of mental processes and a certain invariance, iterative identification in behavior. Psychological defense is a dispositional formation that includes cognitive, emotive and behavioral levels. These levels relate differently to the spheres of consciousness and unconscious: the cognitive aspect presents the logic of consciousness, the emotional aspect – mainly the unconscious perspective through behavior.

Subjectivism generated by protection, on the one hand, allows a person to function normally in society (asserting an idealized "Self"), thanks to the disguise of internal dissociation, inconsistency of the psyche, and on the other – protection generates signs of disintegration, a sense of internal conflict. The study of this angle of protection dynamics allowed T.S. Yatsenko (Yatsenko T.S., Polianychko, O. and Pedchenko, O 2016) to identify previously unknown types of protection – situational and basic (basal).

Basal defenses are associated with the logic of the unconscious, so psychic reality becomes more important than the actual situation of communication. There are distortions that ensure the immutability of the protective mechanisms of the "Self". Basal defenses are formed during the subject's life in a non-experimental way, unique for everyone and filled with infantile drives. Situational protections are aimed at ensuring the social adaptation of the subject. Psychological protection is an integrative formation that masks the internal subject's contradictions.

The task of psychological corrective group work is to reveal the system-forming principles of "psychological defenses" (their basic forms), the awareness of which causes changes in the subject's cognitive, emotional and behavioral spheres. The scientific study of psychological defenses and their functional features in the process of psychological correction involves leveling their situational manifestations and actualization (in dialogue) of basic, basal defenses. This is facilitated by the spontaneity of interaction between members of the group and its humanistic orientation.

The basal defenses that reflect the essence of the psychological correction process are of the greatest interest in the study. Basal defenses can only be learned by identifying the system characteristics of the unconscious that require longitudinal analysis of the subject's behavior over a long period of time. Basal defenses are formed outside of consciousness, on the basis of numerous displacements of certain content of actual experience from the conscious sphere to the unconscious. All this establishes the direction of the psyche, which is determined by its basal defenses.

Deep cognition involves the identification of a logical (associative-figurative) sequence that leads to the deep values of childhood, associated, thanks to fixation, with the focus of energy. The amnesia of childhood experience makes it impossible to reproduce it. Mechanisms developed during the infantile period of psyche formation work on a latent level, but do not lose their influence on the psyche throughout life, masking the infantile significance with the specifics of social situations of the subject. Only certain fragments are consciously reproduced, which in the subject's imagination are difficult to associate with infantile determinants, so their connection with childhood does not lend itself to independent detection and reflection. It is possible to actualize the integral manifestations of the psyche in their systematic order thanks to the professional help of a psychologist. The unconscious, while maintaining its own activity, "makes its way to the surface," however, in a fragmentary and veiled way.

In the context of this problem, it is important to identify relationships that objectify the content of the unconscious. Deep cognition allows to identify a certain fixed infantile content associated with the formation of system characteristics of the unconscious sphere. Of primary importance here is the fact of infantile attraction to parents (Oedipal dependence). And this is understandable, because the first experience of child's emotional contact is received in the family.

Research shows that the subject's psyche depends on family relationships. Contact with the mother is of particular importance – it is always very important in terms of emotional impact, regardless of the gender of the child, because he experiences his first emotional and sensual attraction specifically to his mother. Although the subject is not aware of the significance of sensory contact with the mother, this attraction invisibly contributes to the formation of behavior mechanisms that play a crucial role in determining the subject's expectations of confirmation of his "idealized Self." Against this background, ambivalent feelings for significant people are formed, and thanks to the mechanisms of substitution and transfer, a person cannot get rid of such (formed in childhood) contradiction throughout life. Moreover, the child's relationship with both parents is loaded with primary Oedipal attractions, the manifestation of which in the behavior of different people is individual.

Formed defense mechanisms are "fed" with energy, the direction of which is not given, but is set by ordered fixations of the infantile period of subject's development. This determines the nature of his emotional sphere. Therefore, the psychologist-practitioner should be attentive to spontaneous manifestations of emotions, because they are the first and reliable messengers of the content of the unconscious, which exists outside of time, space and gender.

In the knowledge of the internal characteristics of the psyche, it is important:

- providing the necessary conditions for spontaneous and involuntary behavior;
- practical using of tools for working with the holistic psyche in its conscious and unconscious manifestations;
- knowledge of the relevant theoretical and methodological foundations for understanding the holistic phenomenon of the psyche in its complex relationships, individual uniqueness and inconsistency;
- understanding the dynamics and statics of the holistic phenomenon of the psyche, which is important for understanding its internal features;
- understanding the functional features of the unconscious in the context of consciousness;
- understanding the basic characteristic of the holistic phenomenon of the psyche – its contradictory nature. It is also important to distinguish between types of contradictions: tendencies "to strength" and "to weakness," "to people" and "from people," "to life" and at the same time "to psychological death."

The passage of the future practical psychologist of psychological correction is consonant with the awakening of the instinct of self-preservation. In other words, in-depth training of the future specialist is aimed at forming the prerequisites for practical activity, which anticipates his professional burnout. According to psychodynamic theory, the psychic energy released in connection with the cognition of the unconscious is directed to professional self-realization. The sequence and continuity of the process of personal correction, which turns into self-correction, provide the psychologist with transparency of professional interaction: the inner world of the other becomes clearer, it becomes possible to analyze the current moment in the situation "here and now," to empathize with the emotional state of the other.

Over the past years, the Department of psychology has been conducting groups of personal psychological correction that help students adapt to higher education and allow them to objectivize non-constructive personal formations that complicate the acquisition of the chosen profession. For students of other directions of study, the program of the optional course "Practicum of personal psychological correction" has been developed.

The program of the Practicum provides various methods of work, including conversation, group discussion, role-playing, as well as specific depth-oriented methods – psychoanalysis of non-author's drawing, psychoanalysis of a toy and object model. The participant of the group is presented with a non-author's drawing, he is invited to outline the theme of the drawing, spontaneously and arbitrarily embody himself in any character of the drawing, and express his feelings on his behalf. Working with a non-author's drawing necessarily involves dialogic interaction with the client, as well as the possibility of re-structuring the drawing, adding certain images or ignoring existing ones. The client determines the plot under the influence of his own emotional experiences. Dialogic interaction shows that the images of the drawing, due to projections and identifications of the subject, actualize the emotional aspect of the person. The participants' arbitrary choice of non-author's drawings does not depend on their age, gender, or intellectual characteristics, but is determined primarily by their emotional attractiveness. The results of using this technique confirm its effectiveness in developing the competence of future specialists in the knowledge of the inner world, which implies an understanding of the uniqueness of the deep psychological determinants of one's own psyche through the prism of drawings' symbolism.

The method of working with a toy also proved to be effective. The participant is asked to randomly select a toy from a number of suggested toys, embody the image of the selected model and reveal its attractive characteristics. This type of work makes it possible to approach the spontaneous activity of the client, contributing to the knowledge of the deep tendencies of his psyche.

In deep psychological correction both verbal and nonverbal methods are used. Nonverbal methods rely on nonverbal activity, nonverbal communication and focus on the analysis of nonverbal products. Verbal methods of group work traditionally include group discussion and psychodrama, while nonverbal methods include psychogymnastics, projective drawing, music therapy, etc. This division is quite conditional, since almost any interaction in the group includes both verbal and nonverbal components. Taking into account and analyzing nonverbal behavior (facial expressions, gestures, movements) and interaction in the process of using verbal methods allows to disclose the content of a particular verbal communication more fully and adequately. At the same time, the use of nonverbal means requires verbal interaction in order to get feedback, verbalize nonverbal communication, and emotional state.

Person's capacity to easily take part in different workgroups in spontaneous and previously indefinite situations and calmly deal with it, is the index of the psyche harmony. The emergence of difficulties is due to the presence of internal blocks, resistances. Spontaneity brings to the surface internal determinants that maintain energy potency and rely on fixed, repressed contents. Without spontaneity these problems are invisible, since they are masked by psychological defenses that situationally adapt a person. They play a central role in generating mental dysfunctions: the larger the automated defense system, the more it "comes" from childhood. Defense integrates the psyche, but it does so on a subjective basis, in favor of the idealized "Self," i.e., finds a specific expression in the person's activity and reactions. Therefore, the knowledge of the psyche takes place on the material mediated by the initiative of the protagonist, and not according to a pre-developed plan. "Children's" reactions in adult behavior are an "indicator" of problems in cognition of the psyche.

The head of the psychological correction group pays special attention to impaired perception and reflection of oneself and others caused by the personal problem. The analysis of group material reveals hidden subconscious motives for behavior and choice of psychological specialty, which, under certain conditions, lead to inconsistency of goals and means of achieving them, and as a result, to the emergence of various destructions in relationships with other people.

Such unconscious motives, which are most often identified in the group process, are: an attempt of being the center of attention, a desire for leadership, rejection of weak, insecure people, a tendency to experience their own "strength" at the expense of discrediting others, and so on. It is these unhealthy behavioral tendencies can stimulate the choice of a psychological profession and remain unconscious by the subject himself. When training and performing professional activities, these motives can lead to significant complications of interaction with others, such as the actualization of conflict situations or the emergence of semantic barriers, and will certainly lead to the neurotization of the subject.

Therefore, it is so important to identify students' personal problems with a sense of inferiority or tendencies to psychological death or psychological impotence.

Such people subconsciously try to get psychological help before acquiring professional knowledge and skills in the field of practical psychology. They may be recommended to undergo a repeated psychological correction group in full, which will provide qualified psychological assistance and optimize personal psychological potential.

During deep-correction sessions, external impulses are minimized, because the internally determined rigid tendencies of the personality are manifested. The variety of methods allows to show the subject's features in the most different ways. The subject can be more conscious and mature in the process of professional training after getting this knowledge carried out in the first months of training.

Thus, as a result of passing psychological correction group, students develop important professionally significant skills. In the sphere of communication:

- the capacity to behave spontaneous in a situation of communication with strangers, participate in role-playing games on a given topic;
- the capacity to behave constructively in conflict situations (during a role-playing game);
- the capacity to develop a contact and dialogue with another person in the process of solving a business problem;
- the capacity to feel psychological distance in communication with another person, testing such capacities with other group members;
- the capacity to adequate recognition of the content (meaning) of communication nonverbal means (facial expressions, gestures, pantomimic, etc.).

In the reflexive sphere:

- the capacity to adequate expression of observations, feelings and conclusions about the psychological characteristics of other people and themselves (for example, in the role-playing game);
- the capacity for verbal and vivid expression of the proper emotional experience;

In the emotional sphere:

- the capacity to know emotional responses to another person's unwanted behavior (discontent, irritation, aggression, etc.);
- the capacity to empathize with another person (level of empathy development (on the example of psychodrama));

- the absence of emotional and physical awkwardness, muscle tightness (model of free behavior to music);
- the capacity for expression of actual feelings for other people in a situation of spontaneous relationships.

In the behavioral sphere:

- the basic level of ethical, aesthetic and psychological culture of behavior with strangers and intimate people (building models);
- the capacity for authentic and creative self-expression in telling first impression about the group members;
- the coordination of cognitive and behavioral aspects in self-presentation (on the example of free choice self-presentation form).

REFERENCES

Galushko L., Dmeterko N., Yevtushenko I., Maksimenko E., Pedchenko A., Polyanichko E., Tuz L., Usatenko O. (2012) Psychodynamic Theory: Methodology, Scientific and Practical Achievements. *Psychotherapy*. № 10 (18). Pp. 81–91.

Usatenko O. (2014) Personal Problem of the Subject from the Perspective of Psychodynamic Approach. *Black Sea Scientific Journal of Academic Research*. Tbilisi, Georgia. November. Volume 18. ISSUE 11. Pp. 51–54.

Yacenko, T., Polianychko, O. and Pedchenko, O. (2016) Methodology of Deep Perception of a Person's Mind. *Open Journal of Social Sciences*, 4, 121-127. doi: 10.4236/jss.2016.46013.

CONCLUSION

At the present stage of higher education system development, psychological support of students' professional development is relevant and necessary. It will improve the quality of their training as future specialists. There is a need for a holistic approach to providing psychological support for all participants in the educational process of the University: students, their parents and teachers. The general, integrative criterion of psychological and acmeological development of the students' personality in higher education is the optimality of this process. Optimality refers to the best, in a certain sense, the most favorable interaction between a person and his chosen professional activity. Thus, a fairly high level of professional orientation serves as a criterion for the acmeological development of the individual in early youth. Moreover, this process does not have an end result, but constantly strives for greater awareness, structuring and realization.

Psychological development of the students' personality in higher schools in the educational environment (E. Ponomareva, O. Rudakova), organization of the university psychological service (L. Bura, Y. Zalevskaya), successful adaptation of high school students as a necessary condition for their acmeological development (L. Bura). The process of student adaptation in higher education is a process aimed at achieving a dynamic balance between the student and the educational environment. In this process, the student cannot only adapt and achieve sustainability, but also be able to unlock their potential and make positive changes in the environment.

As a result of an empirical study conducted by S.V. Kucherenko among students of the Pedagogy and Humanities Academy, the features of students' career anchors are clarified. In particular, there was found a low level of orientation to the stability of the place of residence with a high orientation to the stability of the place of work, i.e., a high orientation to building a career in the chosen direction without a desire to work in this region. This may indicate that students and undergraduates of the Pedagogy and Humanities Academy are less likely to seek competence in their careers (Professional competence, Management and Entrepreneurship), while there is an emotional oversupply about the career anchors of needs (Autonomy, Security – the stability of the place of residence and Pure challenge), thus we can talk about an intrapersonal conflict. It can be concluded that the desire to change the place of residence is based on a contradictory desire for autonomy, security and pure challenge. That is, the desire to leave your hometown to build a career in the chosen direction may be related to the manifestation of career anchors' needs, or lack of career anchors of competence. The algorithm proposed in the study allows to design an individual strategy in the field of career anchors of specialists in various fields of training.

According to I.V. Sultanova, a significant part of students with Internet addiction tend to live in the present or yesterday, they have a predominant dissatisfaction with their life in the present and past. Students without Internet addiction are characterized by the presence of certain life orientations, purposefulness, orientation to the present and future. It is also revealed that both groups of students are characterized by fatalism, the belief that a person's life is not subject to conscious control.

Latysheva M.A. suggests using the technology of deep psychological diagnostics in working with first-year students to carry out a comprehensive assessment of personal characteristics and the actual mental state of each of them. The author recommends using these results to develop a program of individual educational route of the student, and, if necessary, to determine the ways of the most effective corrective work at the initial stage of professionalization. Also the basic components of psychological counseling as one of the important areas of work of practical psychologists are analyzed. The review of theoretical sources on the problem of psychological education in the system of psychological support of students in institutions of higher education is presented. It is concluded that psychological education can be effectively implemented only by being integrated into the general system of the educational process at the University. The importance of psychological correction for students of the specialty "Practical psychology" is emphasized, since it is important to identify their personal problems with the presence of tendencies to psychological death, a sense of inferiority and a tendency to psychological damage.

The personal problem is not recognized by the subject, so it is quite difficult to solve it. This is possible with the qualified help of a psychologist who helps to detect the personal problem in its deep psychological essence and transfer it from the implicit level to the explicit one. The subject, as a rule, is aware only of the consequences of having a personal problem (anxiety, tension, increased aggression, etc.), but not its causes. This leads to the fact that many students of the faculty of psychology subconsciously seek rather psychological help, than acquiring professional knowledge and skills in the field. Such people are recommended to undergo psychological correction in full, which optimizes their personal potential.

In addition, psychological counseling (I. Erina), psychological education in the system of psychological support of students (G. Grigoryev) and group variant of deep-correction work in the author's version of T. Yatsenko's psychodynamic approach (O. Usatenko, M. Maik) in the system of higher education of Humanities are disclosed in detail. Psychological education is aimed primarily at the formation of the psychological culture of society in general and students in particular. Thus, the psychological service in education is a practical tool that adapts scientific psychological knowledge to the immediate needs of employees in the field of education and at the same time allows you to solve urgent problems in this area.

ABOUT THE EDITOR

Svitlana Valeriivna Kucherenko, PhD

Born in Yalta, Ukrainian Soviet Socialist Republic (Ukraine). Studied in “Crimean University of Humanities” (Yalta, 1997-2003); Institute of Graduate Education at the V.I. Vernadsky Tauride National University (2003-2005).

Has PhD in Psychological Sciences, “Age and Teaching Psychology” (2011), is Associate professor (2014). Since 2015 works as Associate Professor in the Department of Psychology at the V.I. Vernadsky Crimean Federal University (Yalta, Crimea).

In 2016 she successfully completed the course “Narrative Psychology”. In 2017 she took part in the collective monograph “Development and modernization of pedagogical and psychological sciences: experience of Poland and prospects of Ukraine” (Lublin, Poland).

2019 - professional retraining under the program of additional professional education “Clinical Psychology in Gerontology”.

She is the author of more than 40 scientific articles in the field of personality psychology, narrative analysis and self-awareness of adolescence’s.

ABOUT THE CONTRIBUTORS

Eugene Yurievich Brunner, PhD

V.I. Vernadsky Crimean Federal University

Born in the city of Poltava. PhD (Biology), Associate Professor of Psychology Department.

In 1992 graduated from Simferopol M.V. Frunze State University ("Biologist. Teacher of biology and chemistry". Thesis: "The EHF radiation influence on the pulsed activity of cerebral cortex neurons"). In 2017 graduated from Crimean V.I. Vernadsky Federal University ("Psychologist." Master's thesis: "The specifics of young people attention when working with a proofreading test based on E. Landolt's rings"). In 1997 defended the thesis for the PhD (Biology) degree "Microelectrophysiological investigation of the functional connections between parietal associative cortex and mandibular nerve".

Worked as a senior researcher in the Biophysics laboratories, the Neuronal activity laboratory, the Scientific and Methodological Center for Physical and Physical Health and in the Crimean Research Center, as a programmer in the Center for Vision Rehabilitation, as an inspector in the Crimean Regional Customs, as a psychologist in the Human Rehabilitation Center.

Started teaching in 1999. Gave lectures on psychology in France, Belgium, Latvia, and taught psychology at universities in Ukraine, Russia and China.

Underwent training including advanced training at leading psychologists and practitioners from Ukraine, Russia, France, Belgium, Sweden, Holland, Israel, India in Psychodiagnostic, Psychodrama, Gestalt Therapy, Art Therapy, Fairy Tale Therapy, Hypnosis (classic and Ericksonian), Psychoanalysis, Cognitive-behavioral therapy, Bert Hellinger's Systemic Constellations, Net Work Therapy, NLP, etc. Participated in international TEMPUS-TACIS projects and scientific conferences.

Currently has over 100 publications and a monograph.

Lyudmila Viktorovna Bura, PhD

V.I. Vernadsky Crimean Federal University

Associate Professor, Department of Psychology, Institute of Pedagogy, Psychology and Inclusive Education, Humanitarian and Pedagogical Academy (branch) of FSAEI of HE "Crimean Federal University named after IN AND. Vernadsky" in Yalta.

Academic degree: candidate of Psychological Sciences.

Scientific specialty: 19.00.07 - Pedagogical Psychology.

Education: higher, Voronezh State Pedagogical University, 1999, history teacher; Taurida National University, 2001, practical psychologist.

Sphere of professional interests: management psychology, business communication psychology; Concepts and methods of psychological assistance, mnemonics.

Total work experience: 25 years. Work experience in the specialty: 20 years.

2013 - defense of a dissertation for the degree of candidate of sciences on the topic "Prevention and correction of school maladaptation of primary school students in the process of transition to primary school."

The author of more than 40 scientific papers.

Inobat A. Erina, PhD

Was born in Ganchi (Tajikistan). She graduated from Moscow State Social University. PhD in Psychological Sciences 19.00.05 "Social Psychology" since 2004. Associate Professor since 2009.

Inobat A. Erina is the author of textbooks and scientific articles in social psychology, management and imageology.

Georgiy Pavlovich Grigoriev, MD

Doctor of Medical Sciences, Professor, Professor of the Department of Psychology at the V.I. Vernadsky Crimean Federal University.

In 1964 he graduated Altai State Medical University and in 1996 the Institute of Psychological Culture and Mental Medicine. In 1967 he defended his PhD thesis.

He defended his doctoral dissertation in 1987. For more than twenty years he taught at Altai Medical University. Since 1997 to 2012, he was a Professor at the Yalta University of Management. Since 2012 and still works as an Professor of Psychology at the V.I. Vernadsky Crimean Federal University. Honorary Professor of the Humanitarian and Pedagogical Academy (branch) of the Crimean Federal University.

The author of more than one hundred scientific papers in the field of medicine and psychology.

Marianna Alexandrovna Latysheva, PhD

In 2000 she graduated with honors from the V.I. Vernadsky Taurida National University, faculty of psychology, qualification - psychologist (teaching, scientific work), specialty "Psychology".

2000-2006 – Worked as a school psychologist.

2001 -2006 – Lecturer in the Department of Psychology at the Artek Institute of Humanities.

2006-2014 – Associate Professor, Department of Psychology and Practical Psychology, Crimean Faculty of Humanities, “M.P. Drahomanov National Pedagogical University”.

2005-2008 – Postgraduate studies at the State Educational Institution of Higher Education “University of Education Management” of the Academy of National Economy and Public Administration (Kiev) at the Department of Psychology, specialty 19.00.07 - age and educational psychology.

2008 – Defensed the PhD thesis “Psychological features of the development of intraceptive perception in primary school children”, Kiev, State Educational Institution of Higher Education “University of Education Management” APNU.

2013 – Received the academic title of Associate Professor.

2013 – Awarded with the Honorary Badge of M.P. Dragomanov NPU and Silver medal “Mikhailo Petrovich Dragomanov 1841-1895” for advanced training “Fundamentals of child psychology”.

Since 2015 is Associate Professor, Department of Social Psychology, “V.I. Vernadsky Crimean Federal University”

2015-2016 – Had a professional retraining under the program of additional professional education “Clinical Psychology”.

2020 – Professional development “Fundamentals of child Neuropsychology”.

Maria Stepanovna Maik, PhD

Born in Lviv, Ukraine. In 2006, she graduated from secondary school # 32 of Lviv city and entered the University “Lviv Stavropigion” on the specialty of practical psychology. In 2009, she transferred to the “Crimean University of Humanities” in Yalta to the Department of psychology. In 2011, she received a diploma in social pedagogy and practical psychology. She entered the post-graduate program at the Crimean University of the

Humanities the same year. She defended her thesis and received a PhD in psychology in 2016. Since 2015 she is working as an assistant at the Department of psychology.

Tatiana Pavlovna Pavliuk, PhD

Born in Vinnitsa, Ukraine, studied in "Crimean University of Humanities" (Yalta, 2000-2005); has PhD in philology (Ukrainian language, thesis: The comparison in modern Ukrainian poetry) (2011), is Associate professor (2014). She is the author of textbooks, children's literature and more than 30 scientific articles in the field of syntax and cognitive linguistics.

The range of scientific interests includes the problems of psycholinguistics, sociolinguistics, the functioning of language in the Internet space, and the interpretation of ancient intertexts in French and Ukrainian literature. She is the author of the monograph "Antic Intertext in French Literature of the 20th Century" (2019).

Elena Yuryevna Ponomareva, PhD

Head of the Department of Psychology at the V.I. Vernadsky Crimean Federal University (Yalta, Crimea). Has PhD in Psychological Sciences, 19.00.07 "Age and Teaching Psychology" (2007), is Full professor (2011). Graduated from the Perm Teachers' Institute with a degree in Education and Psychology. Professional interests: psychology of high school, teaching psychology.

Total work experience: 38 years.

Ponomareva E. has more than 100 published educational and scientific works,

Olga A. Rudakova

Senior Lecturer in the Department of Psychology, Chief Specialist in Research and Analysis. In 2010 she graduated from the Crimean Humanities University (Yalta) with a Bachelor's degree in Practical Psychology; in 2011 she graduated from Crimean Humanities University qualified as a specialist in social pedagogy, specialization "Practical Psychologist". Since 2012 in 2016 she is a PhD student in the Department of Psychology in the direction of 19.00.13 – Psychology of Development, Acmeology.

Professional interests: development psychology and acmeology, crisis development psychology, psychological service in educational institutions, psychological diagnosis and personal development. O.A. Rudakova is the author of more than 60 scientific publications.

Olga A. Shutova, PhD

She was born in Lugansk, USSR. In 1998, she went to the Gorlovka State Teaching Training Institute of Foreign Languages.

In 2004 she graduated from the Gorlovka State Teaching Training Institute of Foreign Languages and received a complete higher education in the specialty "Pedagogy and Methods of Secondary Education. Language and literature (English, Russian)" with the qualification of a teacher of English language and foreign literature, Russian language and literature.

From October 2005 to September 2009, she was a graduate student of the Gorlovka State Teaching Training Institute of Foreign Languages. The academic degree of the PhD in Phylological Sciences in the specialty 10.02.15 – general Linguistics was awarded by the dissertation council of the Donetsk National University of the Ministry of Education and Science of Ukraine on February 21, 2011 and approved by the Higher Attestation Commission of Ukraine on May 31, 2011.

Shutova O.A. has 83 published educational and scientific works: 76 – scientific articles and abstracts at scientific conferences, 1 collective monograph, 6 educational and methodological books.

Irina Viktorovna Sultanova, PhD

Head of the Department of Psychology
Sevastopol State University

Born in Sevastopol, USSR.

In 1999, entered the Sevastopol Medical School named after J. Deryugina.

In 2001, entered the Sevastopol City University of Humanities.

In 2004, graduated from the Sevastopol City Humanitarian University and received a complete higher education in the specialty "Psychology" with the qualification of a "Psychologist. Medical psychologist" (specialist, 2004).

From November 2011 to October 2013, she studied in the Crimean University of Humanities.

She has the PhD in Psychological Sciences (specialty 19.00.07–- pedagogical and age-related psychology). The thesis was defensed in the South Ukrainian National Pedagogical University named after K.D. Ushinsky of the Ministry of Education and Science of Ukraine on September 20, 2013 and approved by the Higher Attestation Commission of Ukraine on November 21, 2013.

Sultanova I.V. has 64 published educational and scientific works: 58 - scientific articles and abstracts at scientific conferences, 1 collective monograph, 5 educational and methodological books.

Oksana Nikolayevna Usatenko, PhD

Candidate of Psychological Sciences, Associate Professor of the Department of Psychology at the V.I. Vernadsky Crimean Federal

University (Yalta, Crimea), Head of Research Center of Depth Psychology (Russia). Has PhD in Psychological Sciences, 19.00.07 “Age and Teaching Psychology”.

Professional interests: deep psychology, practical psychology, deep psychological correction of personality and group.

Total work experience: 16 years.

Usatenko O.N. has more than 60 published educational and scientific works and 3 monographs.

Viktor E. Vynohradov, PhD

In 1985 he graduated from the Lviv State Institute of Decorative and Applied Arts. In 2013 he defended his PhD thesis on the topic: "Decorative art in the architectural and spatial environment of Yalta 1880s – 1910s: artistic and stylistic features". The main areas of scientific activity: the exploring the development of decor in the architecture of the modern south coast of Crimea. He is a member of the Union of Designers of Ukraine. V. Vynohradov is the author of more than 30 scientific publications.

Yana Gennadievna Zalevskaya

Assistant in the Department of Psychology at the Humanities and Education Science Academy (Branch) V.I. Vernadsky Crimean Federal University in Yalta. In 2018 she graduated from Humanities and Education Science Academy (Branch) V.I. Vernadsky Crimean Federal University in Yalta, qualification – Master's degree in Psychology, focus program – “Practical Psychology”. Graduate student in the Department of Psychology, direction 19.00.13 – Development Psychology, Acmeology, since 2019.

Her research interests are issues of developmental psychology and acmeology, personal and professional training of future psychologists, depth psychology, theory and practice of deep psychological correction of a personality and a group.

Author of more than 30 scientific articles, including publications in international job.

INDEX

E

F

G

H

I

L

M

Q

R

S

T

U

V

W